The Tabletop
Massage
Manual

MARILYN ASLANI

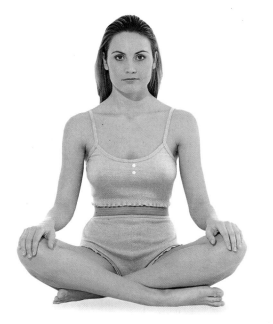

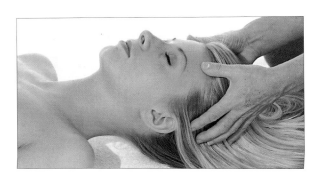

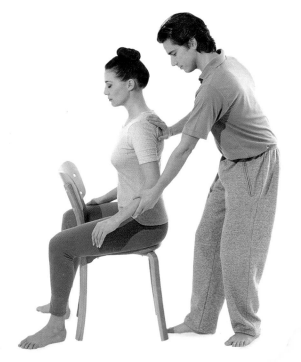

EBURY PRESS
LONDON

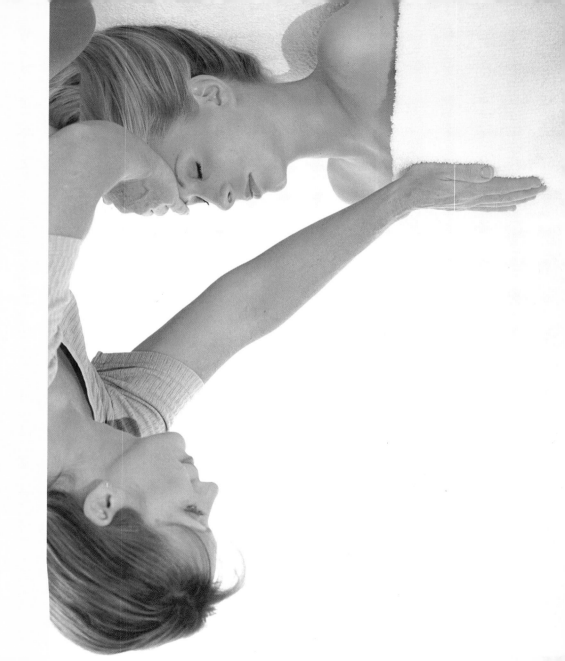

Created and produced by
CARROLL & BROWN LIMITED
5 Lonsdale Road
London NW6 6RA

PUBLISHING DIRECTOR Denis Kennedy
ART DIRECTOR Chrissie Lloyd

EDITOR Sharon Freed

ART EDITOR Lesley Betts

DESIGNER Karen Sawyer

PHOTOGRAPHY Jules Selmes
MEDICAL ILLUSTRATOR Halli Verrinder

PRODUCTION Christine Corton, Wendy Rogers

First published in 1998

1 3 5 7 9 10 8 6 4 2

First published in the United Kingdom in 1998 by Ebury Press
Random House, 20 Vauxhall Bridge Road, London SW1V 2SA

Random House Australia (Pty) Limited
20 Alfred Street, Milsons Point, Sydney,
New South Wales 2061, Australia

Random House New Zealand Limited
18 Poland Road, Glenfield, Auckland 10, New Zealand

Random House South Africa (Pty) Limited
Endulini, 5a Jubilee Road, Parktown 2193, South Africa

Random House UK Limited Reg. No. 954009

A CIP catalogue record for this book is available from the British Library.

ISBN 0 09 186317 1

Printed and bound in Italy by Graphicom

Contents

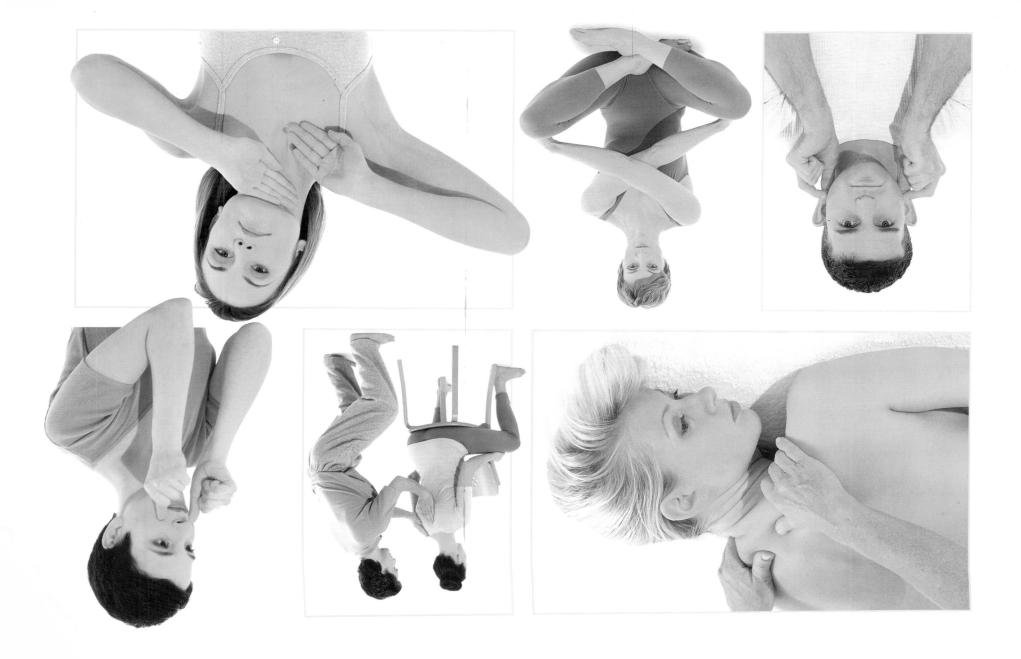

FOREWORD

As the pace of our lives increases within this technological, industrialised age, stress and stress-related disorders are prevalent within our society. In response to this, traditional methods of healing are being rediscovered and their validity recognised. These methods are being used more and more as complements to modern medicine.

Human beings have a deep rooted primal need to touch and be touched. In most instances traditional massage therapies satisfy this need. A connection between giver and receiver is established, resulting in a heightened sense of awareness. During a massage the hypnotic rhythm of the strokes and ensuing relaxation result in a feeling of well-being and calm for both giver and receiver.

Today many people recognise that healing comes from within. We have a part to play in helping ourselves and others towards optimum health.

The Tabletop Massage Manual *enables you to gain the expertise and information to meet some of those needs. Whether you want to help yourself, friends or family, this unique free-standing format will show you how. The flip over pages are filled with photographs clearly illustrating every movement and technique. Detailed instructions for each step are the next best thing to having an expert at your side with individual guidance. Learn to give a full body massage to a partner or to yourself.*

Information for everything that you will need is included from preparing massage oils to professional advice on how and why techniques are performed. You will find out how to bring relief from tension and common ailments, even in the workplace, without the need to disrobe or use oils. Whatever your previous experience or knowledge of massage you will easily learn to effectively relieve tension and common health problems.

It is important to remember to give to ourselves as well as others. Self-care routines are included for simple daily practice, such as the quick energy fix and healing stretches.

I hope that my book contributes to your enjoyment and satisfaction as you acquire new skills which you are able to share with others on a personal level. They are based on my own experience and that of countless teachers and practitioners who for centuries have handed down knowledge which has been followed, adapted and refined, with a common wish of reaching out to one another, to help improve health and well-being.

Marilyn Aslani

HOW TO USE THIS BOOK

This book has been designed with a folding base so that you can stand it up next to you while you massage, without having to hold the pages open. The book begins with an introduction to massage, various massage techniques and preparation for massage. These are numbered from vi to xv and run consecutively. The book then works only in one direction starting with page 1, the beginning of the partnered massage sequence. Stand the book up and flip over the pages, looking only at the lower page. Follow the partnered massage sequence through to page 39. Turn the book around and follow the sitting massage sequence from page 40. On this side of the book you will also find self massage, self energy quick fix, massage remedies for various problems and healing stretches. Again, you will only need to look at the lower pages.

If you have never massaged before, it is advisable that you practise the techniques shown on pages x to xiii until you feel comfortable with them. It may take a while before these movements feel natural. It is important when learning massage techniques that you pay attention to the body you are working on.

To give a relaxing but stimulating massage to a partner follow the complete sequence from page 1 to 39, or to yourself see pages 47 to 59. For a soothing, restful massage omit the percussion techniques (see page xiii). Within the complete massage sequences are separate ones which may be performed individually or in different combinations such as the back, head, face and neck, or feet and hands, depending on what is needed. Make sure if you do one side of the body, such as one foot, that you do the other too in order to maintain balance in the body.

At the top left corner of each partnered massage and self massage pages is a small picture showing what position you need to be in for that page. You will also see the following icons:

Clock This indicates the approximate number of minutes that you should spend on this area of the body. Where you repeat the sequence on the opposite body part, for example the back of the legs, the clock refers to the time required to do both legs. The times given are those recommended if you are following the entire sequence. If, however, you decide just to focus on one area, for instance the back, then you would probably spend a lot longer. The full partnered sequence should take 1–1¾ hours.

Oil Whenever you see this symbol you should oil or re-oil your hands. Never pour oil directly onto the body as it is an unpleasant feeling for your partner. Pour the oil into your hands first, rub them together until the oil is spread evenly and then use long gliding strokes to spread it over the area of the body you are working on. It may take some practice before you get a feel for the correct amount of oil to use. It should enable you to slide easily over the skin but should not be so slippery that you cannot get a good grip on the muscles. Sometimes the word 'optional' appears next to the oil icon. In this case, the technique will work with or without oil.

Hazard This symbol gives you a warning for possible contraindications of massaging this particular area of the body. It is essential that you take heed of these warnings.

Tip Sometimes a handy tip for the masseur will appear and should be taken note of as it will assist you to improve your massage techniques.

Repeat This symbol indicates that you will need to repeat several steps, usually on the other side of the body.

THE BENEFITS OF MASSAGE

The language of touch is universal to humankind. Instinctively we rub aches and pains, or stroke one another to soothe and calm. Massage is one of the earliest techniques used by people to promote good health. There is recorded evidence of massage from many ancient cultures including Egyptian, Greek, Roman, Indian and Japanese. In the early 1800s a Swede, Per Henrik Ling (1776–1839), developed a massage theory, synthesised from Chinese, Egyptian, Greek and Roman techniques, and opened the first institute to offer massage training in Stockholm. This is why massage is often referred to as 'Swedish massage'.

Today the importance of touch therapies is widely recognised. Massage is known to stimulate and regulate physiological processes such as digestion and respiration. It improves muscle tone, joint mobility and postural alignment, enhances the circulation of blood and lymph and balances the hormonal and nervous systems. Not only is massage physically beneficial,

it is psychologically uplifting too – massage conveys caring and acceptance, support and empathy. It helps people to reconnect with their innermost selves and assists in creating a more positive self image. Massage and touch therapies encourage your vital energy or life force to flow freely, restoring your equilibrium and balance.

When giving a massage, always explain to your partner exactly what you are going to do and ask him or her if there are any injuries you should avoid. Stress that during the massage he or she should inform you of any discomfort experienced.

Never massage a person who has any of the following conditions: high temperature, contagious skin conditions, any contagious disease or infection, cardiovascular conditions such as thrombosis or phlebitis. Also, do not massage over varicose veins, recent scar tissue, bruises, tumours, lumps or inflamed joints. If your partner experiences acute back pain which shoots down the arms or the legs during the massage, stop immediately.

If your partner is pregnant, massage very lightly over the abdomen in the first four months. In the remaining months, your partner should lie on her side and massage should still be light and gentle.

AROMATHERAPY

The therapeutic effects of the essential oils have been known for centuries, although the term aromatherapy was only introduced in the 1920s.

Essential oils are known as the life force of aromatic plants and are obtained from their flowers, leaves, stems, bark and roots. When these oils are used in massage, they are absorbed through the skin and bring about a state of harmonious balance and well-being in both the mind and the body. Essential oils can also be used in inhalants, vapourisation, baths, compresses, room sprays and perfumes.

Essential oils fall into the following three classifications:

Top notes: These are the quickest to evaporate and are the most uplifting and stimulating to the body and mind. Examples include bergamot, clary sage, eucalyptus and lemongrass.

Middle notes: Slower to evaporate, these help to improve bodily functions such as digestion and menstruation and include camomile, lavender, rosemary and black pepper.

Base notes: These are the slowest to evaporate and will relax and sedate you. They include sandalwood, jasmine, neroli (orange flower) and ylang ylang.

TOP NOTES

Bergamot	*Clary sage**	*Eucalyptus*	*Lemongrass*
Refreshes, uplifts	Uplifts, warms, relaxes.	Cools body temperature.	Stimulates, cleanses and refreshes
Used for/as: greasy skin, acne, depression, antiseptic, insect repellent	Used for/as: painful menstruation, high blood pressure, astringent.	Used for/as: colds, headaches, asthma, coughs, bronchitis, disinfectant	Used for/as: sore muscles, digestive complaints, acne, antiseptic, astringent.

MIDDLE NOTES

Black pepper	*Geranium*	*Lavender*	*Rosemary**
Warms, stimulates, tones.	Balances, relaxes, stabilises emotions	Balances, restores, soothes, relaxes	Stimulates, revives, improves memory
Used for: muscular aches and pains, toothache, digestive disturbances	Used for/as: depression, menopausal symptoms, neuralgia, astringent, diuretic	Used for/as: insomnia, depression, high blood pressure, digestive disturbances, migraine, nose and throat infections, rheumatism, sprains, acne, bites, boils, sunburn, disinfectant	Used for/as: digestive complaints, respiratory complaints, dandruff, aches and pains, joint pain, disinfectant, diuretic

BASE NOTES

Jasmine*	*Neroli*	*Sandalwood*	*Ylang ylang*
Sensual, relaxes, soothes, uplifts.	Uplifts the spirit, soothes, relaxes	Relaxes, soothes, sensual	Exotic, sensual, soothes, relaxes, uplifts
Used for: skincare, any pain, depression, breathing difficulties	Used for: ageing and blemished skin, anxiety, insomnia, depression	Used for/as: dry skin, acne, coughs and catarrh, nausea, antiseptic	Used for: skincare, anxiety, depression, high blood pressure

viii

Blending oils

Once you have selected appropriate essential oils, they should be added to a carrier oil. Grapeseed is excellent for this purpose as well as being the least expensive. Other suitable oils include soya, sweet almond, peach or avocado. If possible, oils should be 100 per cent unrefined and cold pressed. To preserve your blend add a few drops of wheatgerm oil which is rich in the antioxidant vitamin E.

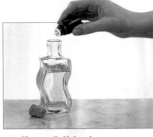

1 For a full body massage use 15 drops essential oil to 30 ml carrier oil.

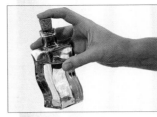

2 Pour the blend into an airtight bottle and store in a cool dark place.

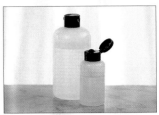

3 A plastic bottle with a flip-top lid is preferable for when you are massaging.

Soothing and relaxing blend

This blend is ideal for stress. tension and insomnia.
5 drops neroli essential oil
3 drops Roman camomile
   essential oil
6 drops lavender essential oil
30 ml carrier oil

Aphrodisiac

This blend is perfect for a romantic massage.
6 drops sandalwood essential oil
4 drops clary sage essential oil
5 drops of either rose, jasmine
   or ylang ylang essential oil
30 ml carrier oil

Blend for aching muscles

Use this blend to relieve and revive aching muscles.
6 drops lavender essential oil
5 drops rosemary essential oil
4 drops black pepper essential oil
30 ml carrier oil

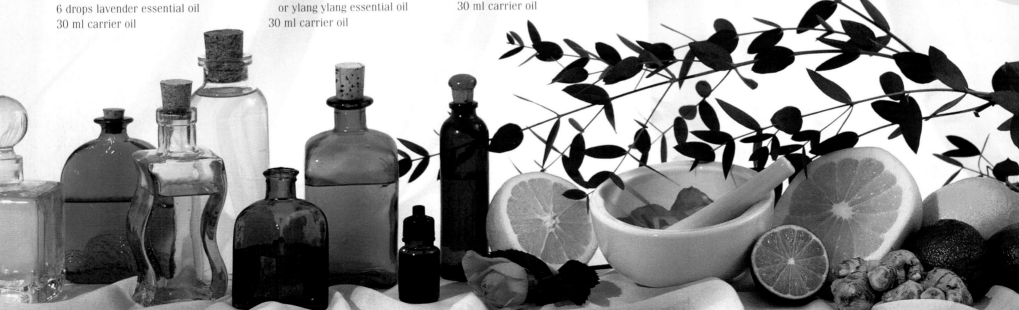

EFFLEURAGE

Effleurage is the name given to the light, soothing strokes which begin and end a massage. They spread the oils and warm the muscles, thereby relaxing them. Effleurage is mainly done with the flat of the hand, keeping the fingers close together. The hands should conform to the natural contours of the body as they slide over it. Effleurage movements should flow without interruption, connecting different stages of the massage. They are normally performed with deeper pressure towards the heart, to aid the venous and lymphatic flow, and with a lighter soothing stroke to return.

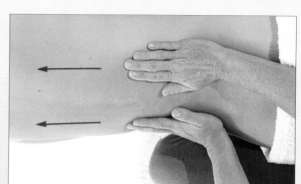

Light stroke

Place both hands flat on the body surface, with your fingers close together, tips slightly raised. In one continuous stroke slide your hands up to the top of the area being worked on, then part your hands and return them back down to their starting position. This stroke should cover as much of the area as possible.

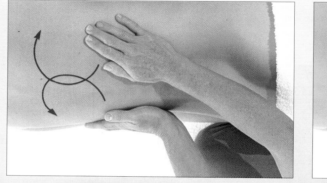

Broad circling

Again keep your hands flat and fingers together and create a swimming motion. Make broad overlapping circles with alternating hands, covering the whole area and reaching down the sides. When you reach the bottom of the area, glide your hands back to the top.

Gliding waves

After using a light stroke up an area of the body, such as the back, move your hands back down in a waving zig zag pattern, bringing them into the middle and out to the sides. Cover as much of the area as possible.

MEDIUM AND DEEP PRESSURE

Any massage should always start off with light strokes, followed by medium and deep pressure, using your thumbs, fingers or the heel of your hands. You also need to learn to apply your body weight to exert more pressure.

Strokes such as thumb circling or thumb rolling are sometimes referred to as petrissage, which is any stroke that grinds the muscles against the bone underneath.

Deep strokes such as petrissage and kneading are stimulating and invigorating, and very effective in improving circulation, eliminating toxins, increasing the metabolic rate, and releasing muscle tension. Thumb circling or thumb rolling can be used on soft tissue over bone but kneading should only be used on very fleshy areas where there is no bone directly beneath it, such as the buttocks. When applying pressure remember that everyone has different tolerance levels, so work gradually and be aware of any reaction from your partner. Avoid using deep pressure techniques over bruised areas or varicose veins.

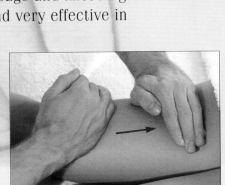

Kneading
With one hand press down on the flesh, and with the other grasp the flesh, picking up the tissue and rolling it away. Release the flesh and grasp it with the other hand, using alternate hands in a rhythmic movement as if you were kneading bread or wringing out a wet cloth. Squeeze and release the flesh with slow movements to avoid just pinching the flesh.

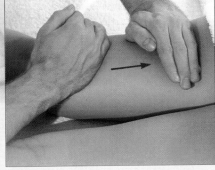

Squeezing
Using the edge of your hand, push into the muscle as you move slowly up it. Your other hand should follow close behind and your hands should keep alternating as they push into the muscle. This can also be done using the heels of your hands, with your fingers pointing upwards. This type of pressure is effective on the front and back of the legs as well as the arms.

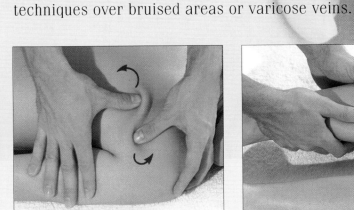

Thumb circling
Use the balls of your thumbs in a circular movement to press and grind the flesh, trapping it against underlying bone. Keep your other fingers relaxed as they follow your thumbs.

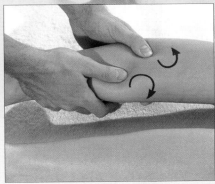

Thumb rolling
Push the flesh away from yourself, using your thumbs in alternating half circles or straight lines in a rhythmic movement. Each thumb is alternately rolling the flesh away from the body. Use your body weight to make the movement deeper. Make the movements slow and firm to avoid tickling your partner.

LYMPHATIC DRAINAGE

The lymphatic system helps to maintain the correct fluid balance in the blood and tissues. Lymph is the vital body fluid between the cells in body tissues. Most of this returns to the blood stream through the capillaries but the remainder is drained into lymphatic vessels where it combines with waste products and micro-organisms such as bacteria. As the fluid passes through these vessels, lymphatic nodes or glands filter off and destroy any disease-causing organisms. Hence the lymphatic system is essential for preventing infections

entering the blood system. The fluid then passes into the veins and is transported back to the heart. Because lymphatic vessels do not pump, lymph can only be moved when muscles surrounding them contract and compress the vessels. This is why both exercise and massage are invaluable for improving lymphatic drainage in the body and in improving the body's ability to fight off disease. The following techniques aid lymphatic drainage from the body tissues back to the heart where the fluid can then be pumped around.

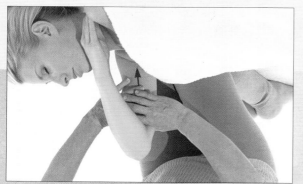

Upper arm

Move closer to your partner's shoulder. With both hands lift her arm at the elbow then bend her forearm so that her hand rests on her opposite shoulder. Now clasp both your thumbs and fingers around the upper arm close to the elbow. Squeeze downwards towards the shoulder. Repeat a few times.

Forearm

Lift your partner's hand so that her forearm is at a right angle. Clasp the fingers and thumbs of both your hands firmly around her wrist. Now squeeze down to your partner's elbow. Bring your hands back to the wrist and repeat a few times.

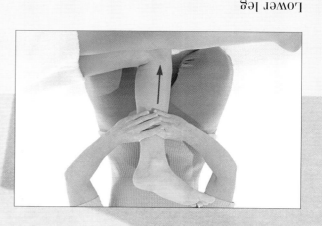

Lower leg

Lift the lower leg with your left hand bringing it back into a right angle. With open thumbs and straight fingers, clasp your hands around the ankle and push them down to the knee, squeezing tightly as you do so. Bring your hands back to the ankle and repeat a few times.

PERCUSSION

These brisk, bouncy strokes are invigorating. They stimulate the blood flow to the skin, thereby improving circulation and waste elimination. They also help to break down fatty tissue and release tension from muscles. Back hand slapping on the upper back helps to decongest the lungs.

The strokes should be kept light and springy rather than heavy or pounding – they should not cause any discomfort. Ask your partner to give you feedback during the massage to ensure that you are performing them correctly.

All these techniques should be performed rapidly with hands alternating to create a rhythmic movement.

They are usually used well into the massage when the muscles have been sufficiently warmed up. If the person being massaged wants to go straight to sleep at the end of the massage do not do these strokes.

Use these strokes on soft fleshy tissue, such as the thighs, buttocks and the tops of the arms. Never use them over any bruises, varicose veins or tender spots.

xiii

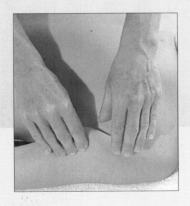 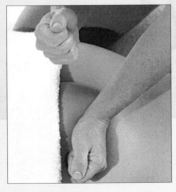 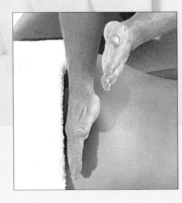 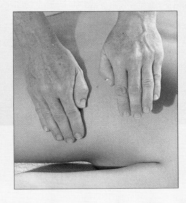 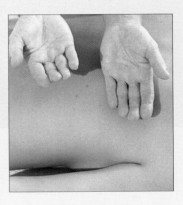

Plucking
With fingers tightly together and hands slightly cupped, pluck and pinch lumps of flesh between your fingers and thumbs.

Pummelling
With loosely clenched fists, use the sides of your hands to drum against the flesh. Let your fists bounce off the flesh.

Hacking
Relax your wrists. With loose fingers, use the sides of your hands to 'karate chop' the flesh. Rapidly bounce your hands off the flesh, one after the other.

Cupping
Draw your fingers and thumbs close together to create a cup shape as if you were going to scoop water to drink. Drum your hands against the skin. When done correctly this creates a vacuum, producing a suction sound.

Back hand slapping
Relax your hands and slap the backs of them lightly against the skin. Keep your fingers and hands loose not rigid.

CREATING THE RIGHT ENVIRONMENT

The surroundings in which you give your massage should contribute to the ultimate relaxation and comfort of both your partner and yourself. Choose a time when you are both free from distractions. Make sure you are not likely to be disturbed during the massage – turn the ringer of the phone down, for instance.

The temperature of the room should be warm enough and free from draughts. As the body temperature tends to drop during the course of a massage, it is wise to have extra towels and a blanket close at hand.

Lighting should be soothing with no overhead or side lights shining directly on to your partner's face. Candles add a relaxing atmosphere to the room, while fresh flowers and an incense or oil burner add fragrance.

The surface on which you work should ideally be a massage table with an adjustable height, but if you are working on the floor, the surface needs to be padded but firm. A carpet with foam rubber or a folded duvet or blanket on top may be used but cover them with towels or old sheets to protect them from the massage oil.

Transfer some oil into a plastic flip top bottle which enables you to control the amount of oil that comes out, as well as avoiding breakages. Otherwise use a small bowl.

Unless your partner finds it intrusive, play soft continuous music to add a relaxing touch, setting the scene for a truly effective treatment.

To start the massage both you and your partner should be relaxed and comfortable. Make sure you are aware of both your own and your partner's posture during the massage.

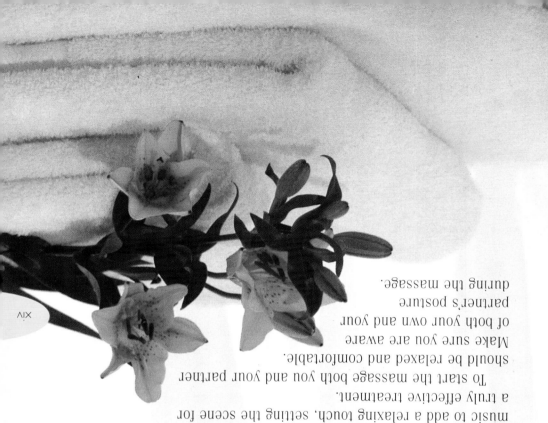

BALANCING YOURSELF

Your own relaxation and comfort are important if you are to give a good massage, either to a partner or yourself. If giving a massage to a partner, wear clothes which are non-restricting. A pair of leggings or tracksuit bottoms are ideal with a short-sleeved, close-fitting t-shirt (a loose one will get in your way)Wear flat shoes or go barefoot.

If you have long hair tie it back. Remove all your jewellery, especially rings, bracelets or watches. Ask your partner to remove all jewellery, glasses, contact lenses and make-up.

To prepare your mind and body before you give a massage you will need to be centred and grounded. Clear your mind of distracting thoughts and focus on the present moment. You need to focus your energy into a central point. When channelled correctly you will become balanced and serene. Relax your belly, your centre, at all times when you work and you will need less muscle power. Your work will become more intuitive and your connection with your partner stronger.

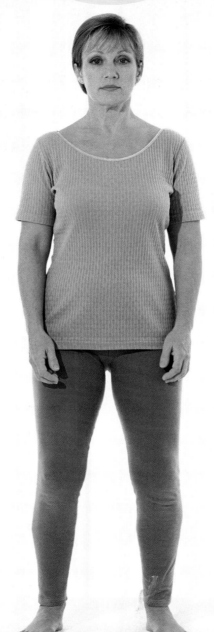

1 The following exercise takes only a few moments and is a *highly effective way of preparing to give a massage.* Stand with your feet a shoulder width apart, facing forwards and knees slightly bent. Keep your spine erect and relax your arms, shoulders and belly. Breathe deeply and evenly. Ground yourself by being aware of your legs and feet solidly on the floor.

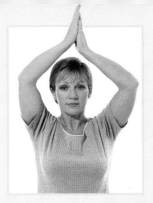

2 Bring your hands up above your head and rub your palms together until they are warm.

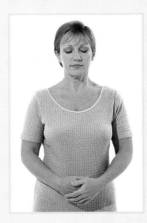

3 Place your hands, one over the other on your belly, below the navel. Close your eyes and concentrate on this area, feeling the warmth from your hands penetrate into your centre. Remain still then slowly open your eyes.

Healing stretches

21 On a carpet or exercise mat, kneel with your bottom on the floor between your feet if possible or, if not, on your heels. Place your hands behind your heels, palms flat on the floor. Lean your body and head backwards and straighten your arms.

22 Lift your pelvis so that you stretch the front of your thighs and body. Stay in this position for a couple of breaths.

23 Lower your pelvis. Bend your arms placing your weight on your elbows. Hold for a couple of breaths. This may be as far as you can go – if so, don't try to push yourself further. Come back to your starting position as you exhale, supporting your body with your hands as you do so.

79

24 If you are able to go down further, breathe in and then, on the next exhalation, lower your body completely on to the floor and bring your arms above your head. Relax for a few breaths and feel the stretch along the front of the thighs, hip and body. If you bring your knees closer together the stretch is more intense. Come back to your starting position in stages as you exhale, supporting your body with your hands.

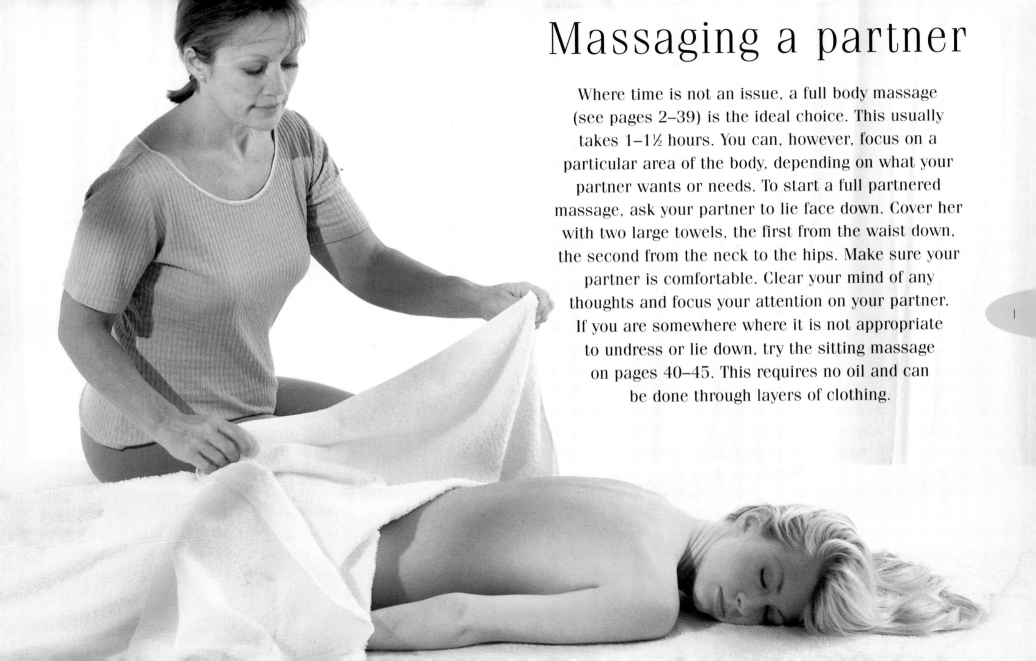

Massaging a partner

Where time is not an issue, a full body massage (see pages 2–39) is the ideal choice. This usually takes 1–1½ hours. You can, however, focus on a particular area of the body, depending on what your partner wants or needs. To start a full partnered massage, ask your partner to lie face down. Cover her with two large towels, the first from the waist down, the second from the neck to the hips. Make sure your partner is comfortable. Clear your mind of any thoughts and focus your attention on your partner. If you are somewhere where it is not appropriate to undress or lie down, try the sitting massage on pages 40–45. This requires no oil and can be done through layers of clothing.

Healing stretches

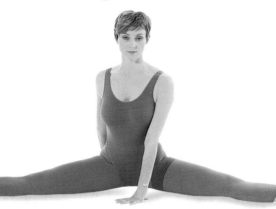

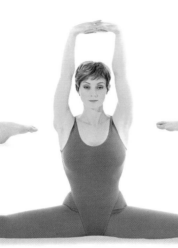

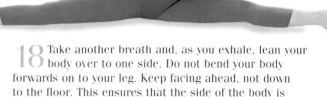

16 Stay sitting on the floor. Open your legs as widely as possible. Place one hand in front of your groin and the other behind you to lift your body forwards, opening your legs even further.

17 Breathe in and stretch your arms up above your head. Interlock your fingers so that your palms stretch upwards.

18 Take another breath and, as you exhale, lean your body over to one side. Do not bend your body forwards on to your leg. Keep facing ahead, not down to the floor. This ensures that the side of the body is stretched as well as the inside of the legs. Hold this position for a few breaths. As you exhale bring your body back up and repeat on the other side.

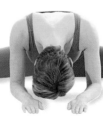

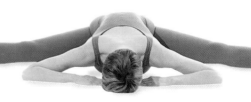

19 Sit up straight then stretch your body out towards the floor. Bend forwards as far as you can, resting your hands, or if possible, your elbows, on the floor. Feel the stretch on the inside of your thighs. Stay in this position for a few cycles of breath, then go to step 20, or sit upright.

20 If you are able to, stretch your body forwards further until you are flat on the floor with arms either stretched out in front or with elbows bent. Stay in this position for a few cycles of breath and then sit upright.

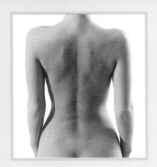

THE BACK

T he best place to begin a massage is the back. For the receiver, this area is like protective armour and less vulnerable than the front of the body. It is also the area of the body which commonly stores the most tension, particularly in the deep and superficial muscles found between and above the shoulder blades, lower back and the buttocks. Massage the muscles in the direction of their fibres (see right). Start with light pressure and gradually increase it as the muscles warm up.

The back is the largest area that you will be working on in terms of size and time, but will afford great pleasure and innumerable benefits to your partner.

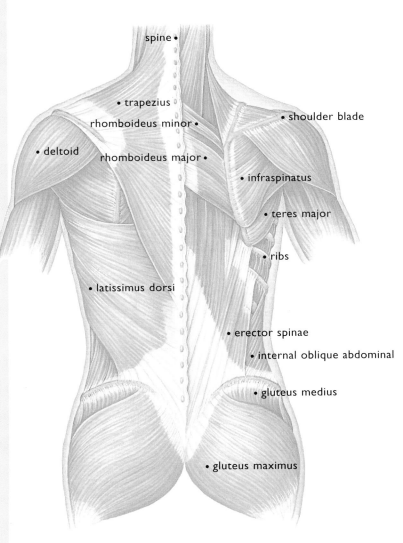

spine •
• trapezius
rhomboideus minor •
• deltoid
rhomboideus major •
• shoulder blade
• infraspinatus
• teres major
• ribs
• latissimus dorsi
• erector spinae
• internal oblique abdominal
• gluteus medius
• gluteus maximus

◄ **The spine**
This is made up of 24 vertebrae (small bones) separated by pads of fibrocartilage. Do not massage over the vertebrae.

◄ **The shoulder blades**
There are many muscles attached to the shoulder blades which often store tension. You can use pressure over them.

◄ **The spinal cord**
This runs down through the spine. Nerves which branch out through the vertebrae link the brain to other parts of the body. By massaging either side of the spine, you will be balancing the nervous system.

◄ **The sacrum and coccyx**
These are fused, immobile bones at the base of the spine. You can use some pressure over the sacrum unless your partner has a lower back injury.

◄ **The kidneys**
These are positioned against the back of the abdominal wall at the waist line on either side of the spine. Always use light pressure when working over this area.

◄ **The buttocks**
Deep pressure may be used on the gluteal muscles which cover the buttocks.

Note: The left side of the diagram shows superficial muscles and the right side deep muscles.

2

Healing stretches

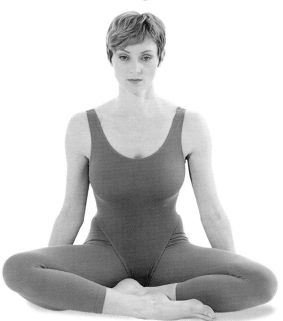

13 Still in a sitting position, cross your legs, bringing your right foot in front of the left. Straighten your back.

14 Raise your knees. Bring your right arm to the front, and place your hands on the outside of your thighs, just above the knees.

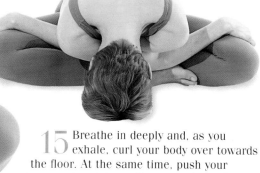

15 Breathe in deeply and, as you exhale, curl your body over towards the floor. At the same time, push your knees out and down. Keep your buttocks firmly on the floor. Feel the stretch in between your shoulder blades, as well as in your back and hips. Stay down for another couple of breaths. Come up as you exhale. Change your position so that your left leg and arm are in front. ◁◁ Repeat steps 13 to 15.

The back

 Take your time to relax and connect with the body before massaging

1 Place your right hand on your partner's lower back and your left hand on the upper back. Close your eyes and breathe deeply. Focus your attention on your hands and relax.

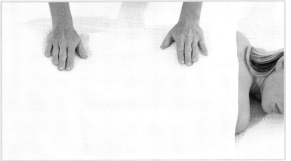

2 Now move your right hand to the side of your partner's left buttock, leaving your other hand on the upper back. With minimal force, begin to rock using the heel of your hand to gently push your partner's body away from you.

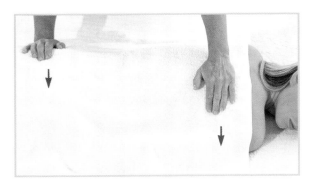

3 Continue rocking as you bring your left hand next to your right. Rock gently.

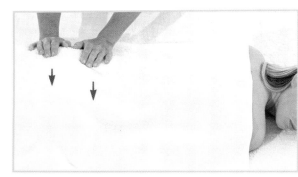

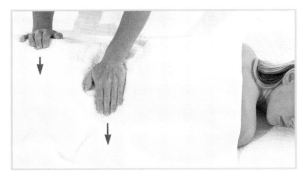

4 Still rocking the body, gradually move your left hand along the entire back – first up the left side then down the right. Slowly bring the rocking to a close.

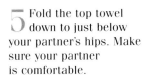

5 Fold the top towel down to just below your partner's hips. Make sure your partner is comfortable.

3

Healing stretches

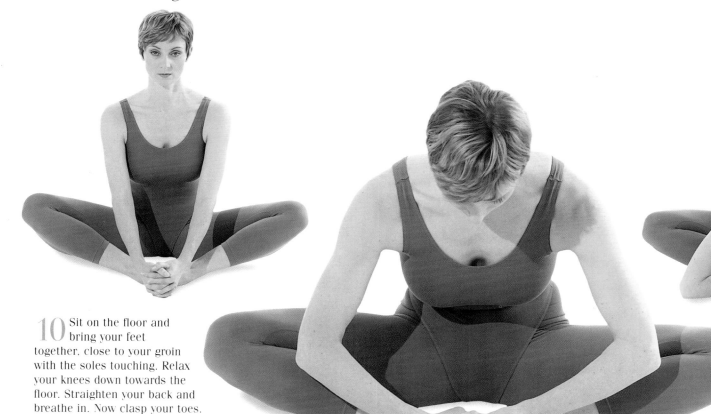

10 Sit on the floor and bring your feet together, close to your groin with the soles touching. Relax your knees down towards the floor. Straighten your back and breathe in. Now clasp your toes.

11 As you exhale relax your head and body and bend forwards. Keep your buttocks firmly on the floor, as you bring your head down towards your feet. Allow your elbows to relax towards the floor.

12 Stay in this position for another four breaths. Each time you exhale, curl your body over, so that your head and elbows sink lower. At the same time, push your knees outwards and down towards the floor. Feel the stretch across your shoulders and down your arms, as well as in your back and groin. Breathe in, then curl up slowly on the outbreath.

76

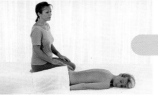

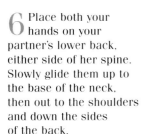

The back

 Avoid using pressure over kidney area

 Increase the depth of your pressure gradually as the back warms up

6 Place both your hands on your partner's lower back, either side of her spine. Slowly glide them up to the base of the neck, then out to the shoulders and down the sides of the back.

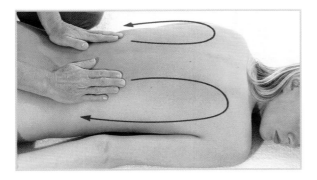

7 As you glide back down to the waist, pull upwards and inwards. ◁◁ Repeat steps 6 and 7 until the back is well oiled and it feels warm.

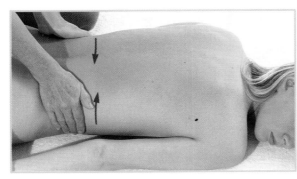

8 Starting at the lower back, use a swimming motion to make broad over-lapping circles with your hands on either side of the back. Move up towards the shoulders and straight back down the sides. Repeat several times.

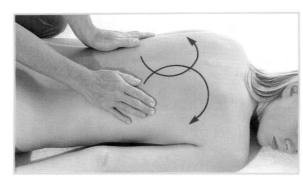

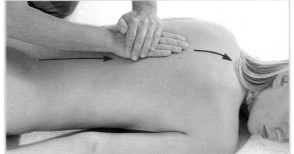

9 Place your right hand at the base of the spine, with your fingers pointing towards your partner's head. Lay your left hand across it and glide your reinforced hand up to the neck.

10 Remove your left hand and use your right index and middle fingers to press down on either side of the spine. Alternate with your left hand and work down to the lower back.

4

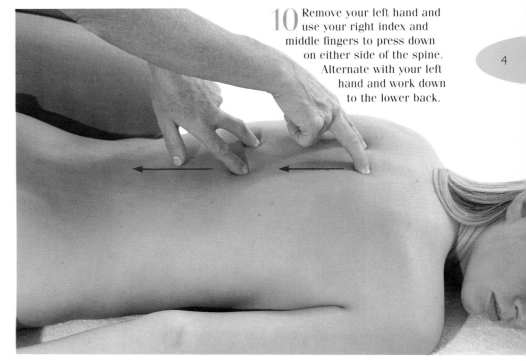

◁◁ Repeat steps 9–10. Then move your position slightly up the body and facing in.

Healing stretches

4 Sit on the floor with your feet stretched out in front of you.

5 Breathe in as you bring your hands up above your head, with the palms facing outwards. Pull up, stretching the length of your spine.

6 Exhale as you slowly bend forwards, bringing your arms down to shoulder level and reaching to touch your feet. Keep your back and legs straight, look straight ahead.

7 Inhale deeply, and on the exhalation, bend forwards trying to stretch your hands beyond your feet.

8 Breathe in again, then relax your body and head down on to your legs if you are flexible enough. Stay down for a couple of breaths. If you can't, go to step 9.

9 As you breathe out slowly uncurl your back and head and return to an upright position.

75

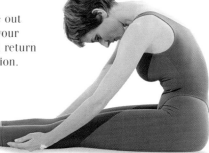

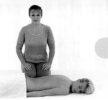

The back

Avoid using pressure over kidney area

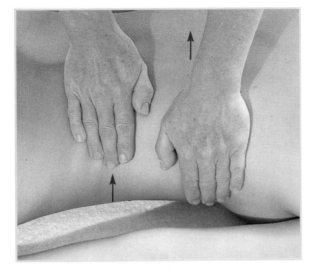

Very deep pressure should only be used over fleshy areas of the body

11 Starting at the buttocks, use alternate palms to pull up from the sides, following the curves of the body. At the top, pull your fingers across the shoulder towards the neck. Then work back to the lower hip. The hands should follow each other closely so that contact with the body is not broken.

13 Knead the flesh of the buttocks. Use alternating hands to grasp and squeeze the flesh, gradually increasing the pressure. Move up the back, then knead the top of the arm. Roll the flesh of the shoulder between your thumbs and index fingers. Lightly knead the back of the neck. Move down between the spine and shoulder blade.

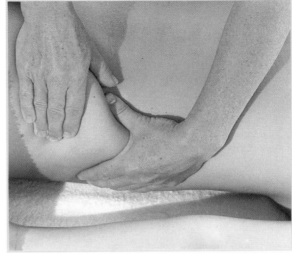

5

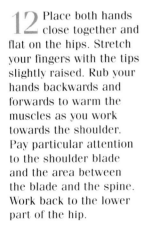

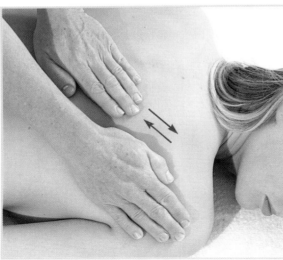

12 Place both hands close together and flat on the hips. Stretch your fingers with the tips slightly raised. Rub your hands backwards and forwards to warm the muscles as you work towards the shoulder. Pay particular attention to the shoulder blade and the area between the blade and the spine. Work back to the lower part of the hip.

14 Working from the spine towards the blade, roll your thumbs in alternating outward circles. Ask your partner for feedback as you increase the pressure into these muscles. In most instances, this technique produces a 'pleasant pain' and a welcome sensation of tension being relieved. Work across the shoulder blade.

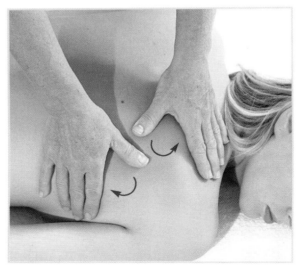

Now knead back down to the buttocks.

Healing stretches

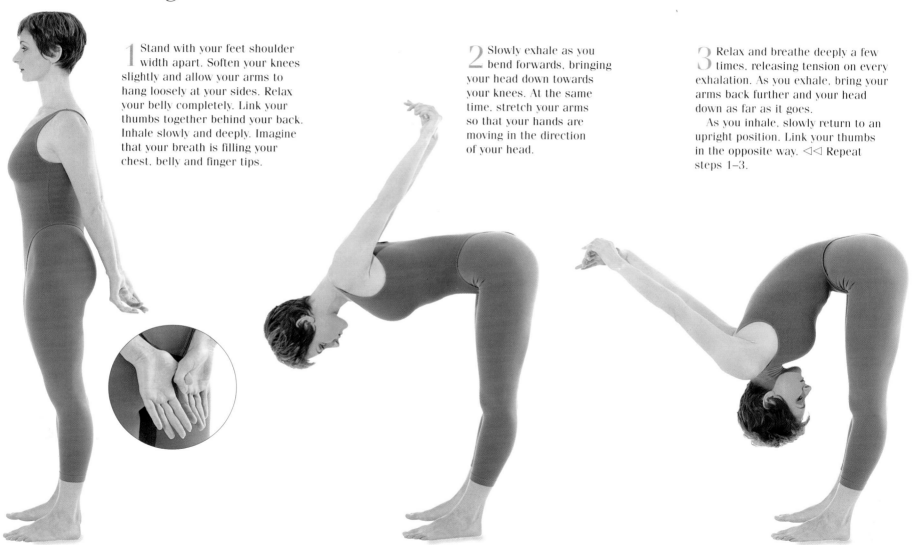

1 Stand with your feet shoulder width apart. Soften your knees slightly and allow your arms to hang loosely at your sides. Relax your belly completely. Link your thumbs together behind your back. Inhale slowly and deeply. Imagine that your breath is filling your chest, belly and finger tips.

2 Slowly exhale as you bend forwards, bringing your head down towards your knees. At the same time, stretch your arms so that your hands are moving in the direction of your head.

3 Relax and breathe deeply a few times, releasing tension on every exhalation. As you exhale, bring your arms back further and your head down as far as it goes.

As you inhale, slowly return to an upright position. Link your thumbs in the opposite way. ◁◁ Repeat steps 1–3.

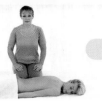

The back

Avoid using pressure over kidney area

15 With your palms together, rest your forearms across the centre of your partner's back.

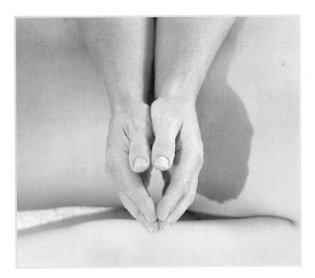

16 Slowly push your arms apart in opposite directions, rolling your arms so that your palms face down. Your right arm should stop at the base of the spine and your left arm at the top of the neck. Use your body weight to apply pressure.

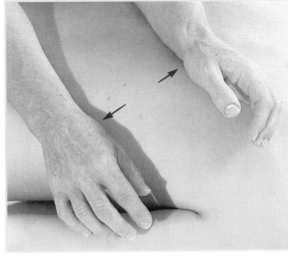

17 Now repeat this movement diagonally on both sides. Your left arm should slide up to the shoulder, while your right arm slides off the opposite buttock.

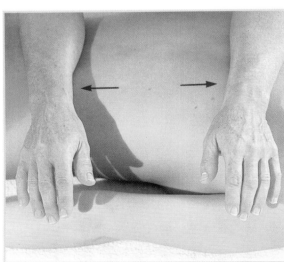

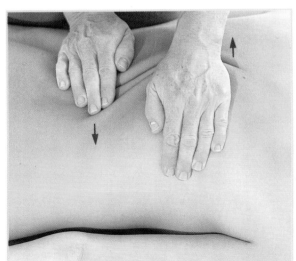

18 Place both hands in the same direction on the buttocks and use a criss-cross, wringing motion to move up the back. As you push forwards with one hand, pull backwards with the other, using the heels and fingers of both your hands against the back. Keep your hands moving in alternate directions.

6

Move to the right side of your partner. ◁◁ Repeat steps 11–18 on the right side of the back.

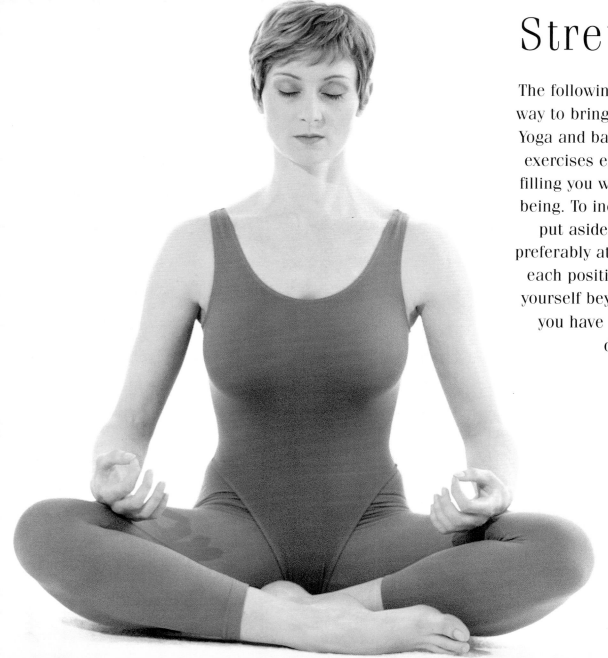

Stretching yourself

The following healing stretch routine is an excellent way to bring your body back into balance. Similar to Yoga and based on ancient oriental practices, these exercises encourage blocked energy to flow freely, filling you with renewed vigour and a sense of well-being. To increase your flexibility and vitality, try to put aside ten minutes per day for this routine, preferably at least two hours after eating. Relax into each position as you breathe out without pushing yourself beyond what is comfortable for you. When you have completed them, sit still and breathe deeply, focusing your energy.

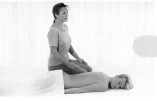

The back

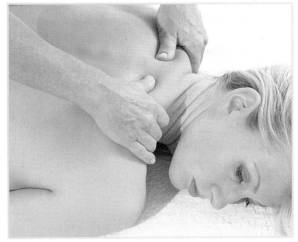

19 Move back to the left side of your partner. Slide both your hands over the tops of each shoulder. Knead the shoulders and base of the neck lightly, squeezing and 'rolling' the flesh between your thumbs and fingers.

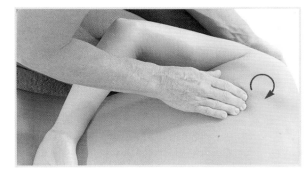

21 Place your left hand under your partner's left shoulder. With your fingers together and using circular movements, massage all over the shoulder blade and the muscles between it and the spine.

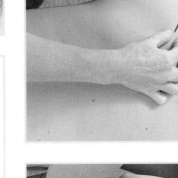

22 Find the bony ridge that runs across the top section of the shoulder blade. From the neck, in an outwards direction, squeeze the flesh along the ridge between your thumb and fingers.

7

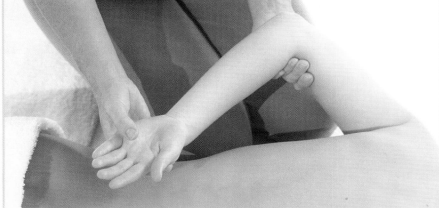

20 Bring your left hand down to your partner's left elbow. With your right hand pick up your partner's hand. Now bend the elbow and lift the forearm across the back and rest it there.

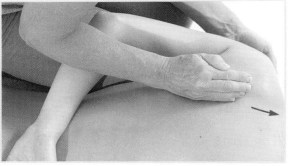

23 With fingers together, place the side of your hand at the inside top of the blade. Lift the shoulder slightly and slide your hand down underneath the blade. ◁◁ Repeat steps 21–23.

Move to the right side of the body. ◁◁ Repeat steps 20–23 on the right shoulder.

Sports injuries

Massage is highly recommended before and after exercise. Before exercise use invigorating techniques such as kneading and percussion (see pages xi and xiii). After exercise use lymphatic drainage and deep tissue techniques (see pages xi and xii) to help eliminate waste products that have accumulated in the muscles. Massage is also very effective in treating sports injuries.

A muscle cramp results from restricted blood flow to that area. Massage can help to improve circulation and bring relief. For a leg

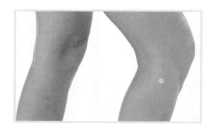

cramp, lie down and raise the leg. Then sit up and stroke the whole leg, towards the body, then knead the muscles which are cramped.

Muscle strains and sprains result when a muscle is placed under prolonged stress such as excessive exercise, or twisting or wrenching movements which stretch the ligaments connecting bone to muscle until it tears. The soft tissue surrounding the area then becomes swollen, bruised and very painful.

If you suspect you have strained or sprained a muscle or ligament, use cold compresses or packs, or even a packet of frozen peas over the area, to reduce swelling or inflammation. Keep the limb

elevated. See a doctor immediately to rule out the possibility of a fracture or broken bone. If a sprain or strain is confirmed, massage gently around the injury, with upward movements, to help drain fluids.

Depending on your injury, apply pressure to the following points for 3–7 seconds.

> *To relax tendons, muscles and joints:*
> Press points 1 and 3
> *For swelling in the lower leg:* Press point 2
> *For cramp in the lower leg:* Press point 4

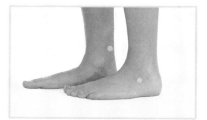

● *Point 1*: In the depression below the head of the fibula bone.

● *Point 2*: Two thumb widths above the tip of the inside ankle and the Achilles tendon.

● *Point 3*: In the depression below and in front of the outer ankle.

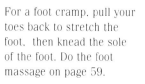

For a foot cramp, pull your toes back to stretch the foot, then knead the sole of the foot. Do the foot massage on page 59.

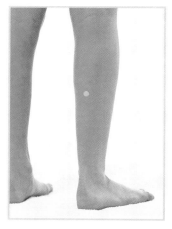

● *Point 4*: In the centre of back of the calf, between the knee and the ankle. Press until the cramp subsides.

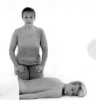

The back

Use only light pressure over the kidney areas

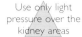

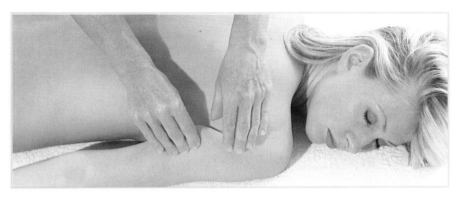

24 Move back to the left side of your partner and work on the right side of the back. Working from the buttocks up to the shoulders and tops of the arms, pluck and pinch lumps of flesh between your fingers and thumbs.

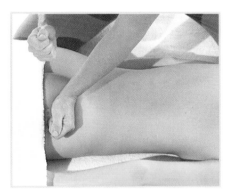

25 With loosely clenched fists, use both your hands to pummel against the right buttock.

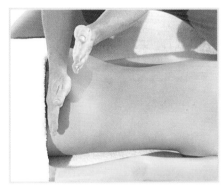

26 With loose fingers, and palms facing each other, use the sides of your hands to hack the buttocks rapidly.

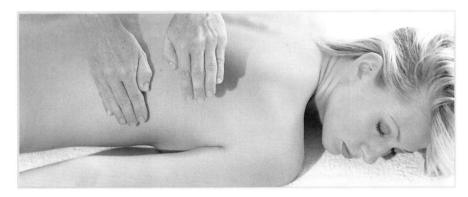

27 Create a cup shape with your hands. Start at the buttocks and drum your hands against the skin. When done correctly, this creates a vacuum, producing a suction sound. Work up the whole of the right side of the back and include the top of the arm.

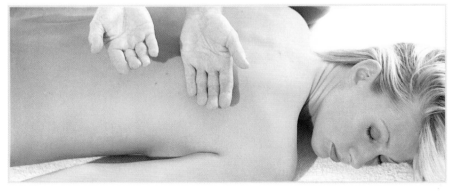

28 Starting at the buttocks again, relax your hands and slap the backs of them lightly against the skin. Use this technique over the entire right side of the back and upper arm.

Move to your partner's right side. ◁◁ Repeat steps 24–28. Then move to sit at the head.

Coughs and asthma

Asthma is caused by spasms in the muscles surrounding the bronchii, constricting the outward passage of air. Coughing, wheezing and tightness in the chest are all symptoms and breathing can be difficult. Dry towel massage can be beneficial for coughs, asthma and colds.

Several pressure points along the arms and on the chest clear heat from the lungs, which can bring relief to those suffering with coughs or asthma. Take a dry towel and rub the arms and legs towards the heart. Continue until the body feels warm. This promotes good circulation and skin respiration, improving the health of the whole body.

Either ask someone to give you a chest and arm massage (see pages 32 and 27–29) or follow the self massage sequence (pages 52–53).

Use any of the following oils:
Asthma: cypress, camomile, cajput, bergamot (do not use oils in steam inhalation for asthma).
Coughs: benzoin, cajput, cedarwood, marjoram, tea tree.

During the massage apply pressure to the following points, pressing each for 3–7 seconds.

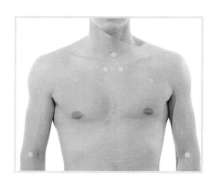

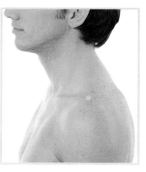

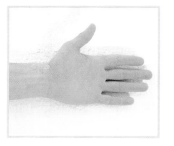

- *Point 1*: In the centre of the base of the throat.
- *Point 2*: Below the mid-end of the collarbone.
- *Point 3*: On the breast bone between the nipples.
- *Point 4*: Below the first rib above the nipple.
- *Point 5*: In the elbow crease on the thumb side of the tendon.

- *Point 6*: On top of the shoulder where the collarbone and shoulder blade meet.

- *Point 7*: One and a half thumb widths from the wrist crease below the base of the thumb.
- *Point 8*: Below the wrist crease under the base of the thumb where a small pulse can be felt.

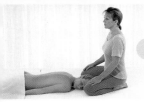

The back

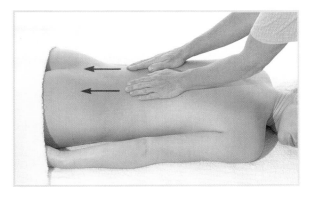

29 Gently place your hands on either side of the spine, with fingers pointing towards the feet. Slowly glide them from the neck down to the base of the spine, using your body weight as you move down.

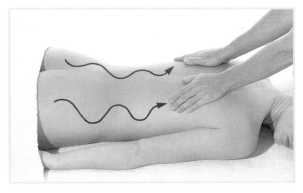

30 From the base, use the heels of your hands to create a waving zigzag pattern all the way up the back, moving out towards the sides, then in towards the spine.

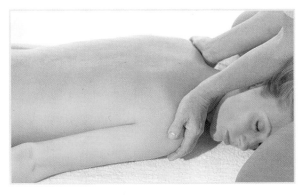

31 Continue these gliding waves over the tops of your partner's shoulders, reaching underneath them as your hands move towards the neck.

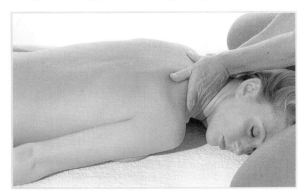

32 Now bring your hands in and squeeze gently up the sides of the neck. Bring your fingers to rest under the bony ridge at the base of the skull, and press into this ridge.

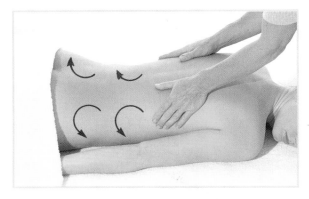

33 Place your hands on either side of the spine at the shoulders. Form broad outward circles with your hands and circle your thumbs in the same direction, pushing them into the muscles. Work down the back with firm pressure.

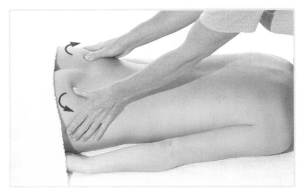

34 Using the same technique, push the thumbs into the muscles at the top of the buttocks and out to the sides. Return to the shoulders with a long gliding wave and finish with a neck squeeze.

Menstrual problems

Massage can help to relieve the symptoms of Premenstrual Syndrome (PMS) and menopause.

These can include depression, cramps, water retention, headaches, backaches, insomnia and emotional stress. A soothing massage helps to bring the body back into a state of calm and balance. A complete body massage is best but if the abdomen is sore and time is limited, work on the lower back and legs.

If you are being massaged ask your partner to follow the routines on pages 2–10 and 12–19. If you are massaging yourself, follow the routines on pages 51 and 56–58. During the massage the following points should be incorporated. Or, if you are short of time, simply press into these points for 7–10 seconds each.

The following essential oils can enhance the therapeutic effect of your massage. Add them to your base massage oil:
For all menstrual problems – rose
For scant and irregular periods – jasmine
For heavy periods – frankincense
For cramping pain – marjoram
For menopause and to balance hormones – geranium

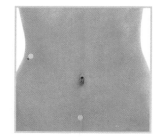

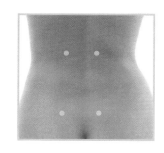

● *Point 1:* Two thumb widths above the pubic bone on the midline of the body.
● *Point 2:* At the end of free end of the twelfth rib.

● *Point 3:* One and a half thumb widths either side of the spine, at the level of the second lumbar vertebra.
● *Point 4:* Either side of the base of the sacrum.

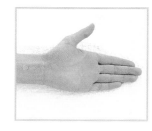

● *Point 5:* Two thumb widths from the wrist crease in between the two tendons.

● *Point 6:* Four finger widths above the inner ankle under the tibia bone.
● *Point 7:* Two thumb widths above the inner edge of the knee.

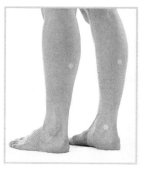

● *Point 8:* In the centre of the calf halfway between the knee and the ankle.
● *Point 9:* Between the inner ankle and the Achilles tendon.
● *Point 10:* Between the outer ankle and the Achilles tendon.

70

The back

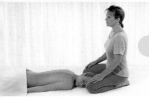

35 Stretch your fingers and thumbs into a V-shape and place them either side of the spine. Starting at the shoulders, push down on the muscles as if flattening them. Use a long gliding stroke back to the head.

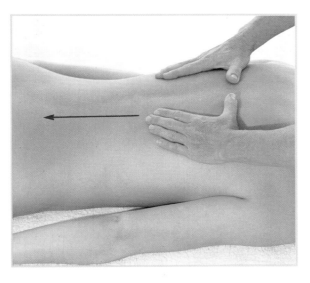

36 Start at the base of the neck and work downwards on either side of the spine. Using your thumbs, make small outward circular movements. Keep fingers relaxed. Use fairly deep pressure at the top of the back, gradually decreasing as you descend. Use a gliding wave to return upwards.

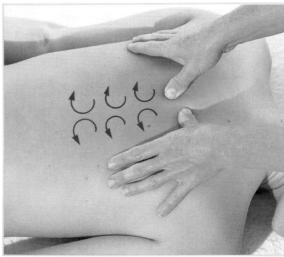

37 Place both hands flat on your partner's shoulders. Using your hands alternately make broad circles down the whole of the back and then cover the buttocks.

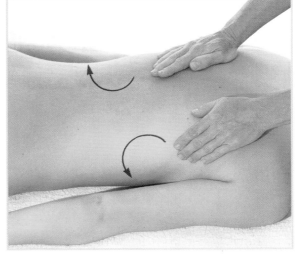

38 Starting at the base of the spine use the tips of your fingers, as if playing the strings of a harp, to caress gently up the whole back. At the shoulders bring your hands in, so that this 'feathering' includes the neck. Brush over the top of the head.

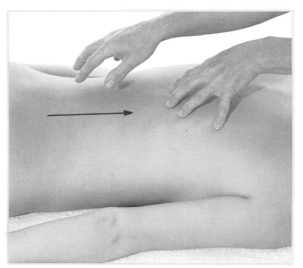

10

Cover your partner's back with the towel. Move down to the feet.

Constipation

Constipation usually arises from insufficient amounts of fibre and fluids in the diet, and results when waste material moves too slowly through the large bowel. Some other causes are pregnancy, lack of exercise, nervous tension, stress and the side effects of some drugs.

Elimination of wastes should take place every 18 to 24 hours, after this harmful toxins spread through the body and side effects such as headaches, skin blemishes, insomnia, bad breath and indigestion may follow.

Natural laxatives such as prunes, figs and linseed or castor oil can be taken. Half a cup (125 ml) of aloe vera juice in the morning and at night are beneficial and fresh fruits and raw green leafy vegetables should be eaten on a daily basis.

Follow the instructions for the abdomen massage (page 31 or 55), paying particular attention to the left side, the area of the descending colon. Always massage the abdomen in a clockwise direction only.

Cardamom oil is refreshing, invigorating and warming. It should be massaged on the abdomen for digestive complaints. Coriander and fennel are also beneficial. Apply pressure for 3–7 seconds to the following points.

Avoid pressing point 8 if you are pregnant.

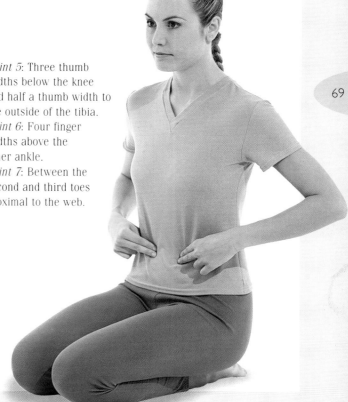

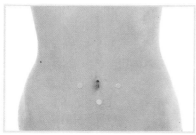

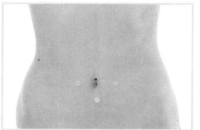

- *Point 1*: Two thumb widths either side of the navel.
- *Point 2*: One and a half thumb widths below the navel.

The area of the descending colon should also be massaged with the thumb and fingers and kneaded. This is on the left side of the abdomen.

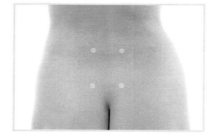

- *Point 3*: One and a half thumb widths on either side of the spine level with the fourth lumbar vertebra.
- *Point 4*: On either side of the spine in the first sacral notch.

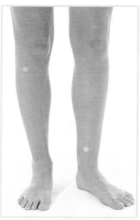

- *Point 5*: Three thumb widths below the knee and half a thumb width to the outside of the tibia.
- *Point 6*: Four finger widths above the inner ankle.
- *Point 7*: Between the second and third toes proximal to the web.

69

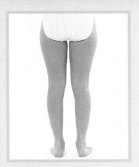

BACK OF THE LEGS

Massaging the large fleshy muscles at the back of the legs improves circulation and lymphatic drainage as well as helping to prevent varicose veins and swelling in the lower legs.

As you work, gradually increase the pressure into all of these muscles to relieve tension. Always use stronger pressure on the upward strokes to aid the flow of blood returning to the heart.

If any varicose veins are present, brush your hands over them with the lightest touch possible. Never apply any pressure over them.

When stretching the front of the thighs and the feet, do so with care, avoiding sudden jerky movements.

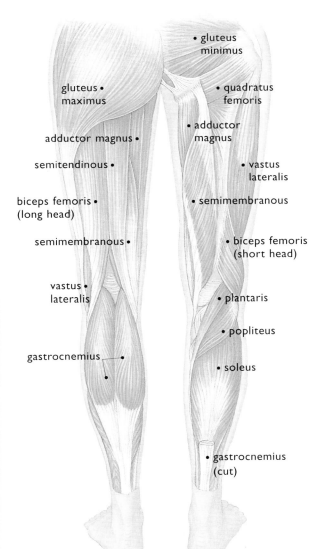

gluteus minimus

gluteus maximus

quadratus femoris

adductor magnus

adductor magnus

semitendinous

vastus lateralis

biceps femoris (long head)

semimembranous

semimembranous

biceps femoris (short head)

vastus lateralis

plantaris

popliteus

gastrocnemius

soleus

gastrocnemius (cut)

◄ The sciatic nerve

This nerve, which is about the same diameter as your thumb, runs down the back of the thigh before it divides at the knee and branches down the calf and foot. If your partner suffers from sciatic pain in the lower back and leg, she will get great relief from having her legs massaged.

◄ The hamstrings

These muscles (biceps femoris, semitendinous and semimembranous) at the back of the thigh are the most likely to get stiff after vigorous exercising and should be stretched before and after exercise.

◄ The back of the knee

The area at the back of the knee is soft and vulnerable and should only be worked on with the lightest touch. Avoid using any percussion techniques on this area.

◄ The soleus and gastrocnemius

These muscles at the back of the lower leg are often tight and tender. As you work upwards, press into the centre of the muscle, as if separating it. To relieve cramp in these muscles, press into the midpoint of the calf between the back of the knee and ankle for approximately ten seconds.

Note: Superficial muscles are shown on the left leg and deep muscles on the right leg.

11

Lower back pain

Millions of people suffer from lower back pain which can be caused by being overweight, lack of exercise leading to weak leg and back muscles, sleeping on soft beds or bad posture.

Prevention is far better than cure, but if you are already in pain the following should be helpful, as long as you have seen a doctor and have no broken bones, slipped discs, bone diseases or other serious bone problems.

Rest and stay quiet. Lie on a firm mattress in a comfortable position. Keep your back warm with hot water bottles or towels to promote blood circulation.

If someone can give you a massage, ask him or her to follow the back and back of leg sequences on pages 3–15, or if you can comfortably do so, follow the self massage on pages 51, 56–59. Use warming oils such as black pepper, cardamom or cinnamon. Incorporate the following pressure points into your massage and press for 3–7 seconds during the course of your massage.

Avoid pressing point 8 if you are pregnant.

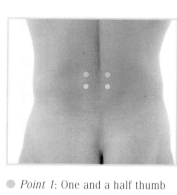

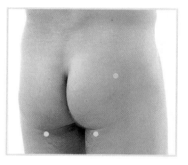

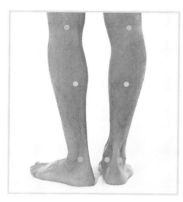

- *Point 1*: One and a half thumb widths on either side of the spine at the level of the second lumbar vertebra.
- *Point 2*: One and a half thumb widths on either side of the spine at the level of the fourth lumbar vertebra.
- *Point 3*: On either side of the spine in the second notch of the bony triangle.

- *Point 4*: In the main depression at the side of the buttocks.
- *Point 5*: In the mid-point below the crease of the buttock at the top of the thigh.

- *Point 6*: In the centre of the back of the knee.
- *Point 7*: In the centre of the calf, midway between the back of the knee and the ankle.
- *Point 8*: Midway between the outer ankle and Achilles tendon.
- *Point 9*: Midway between the inner ankle and Achilles tendon.

Back of the legs

   Avoid massaging over varicose veins If your partner is cold, cover the leg that you are not working on

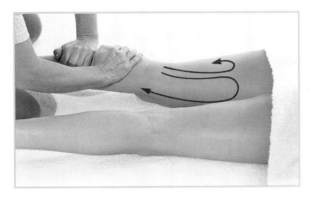

1 Rest your hands across the back of the left ankle. Push both hands up to the top of the thigh, part them and gently return down, one hand on each side, following the contours of the leg. Repeat.

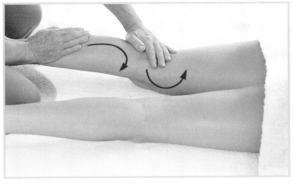

2 Starting at the ankles, make overlapping oval shapes, moving upwards about 2.5 cm at a time to the top of the leg – one hand following the other. Gently glide back down the sides to the ankles.

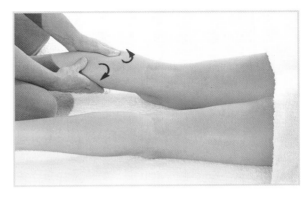

3 Work up the calf to the base of the knee, using your thumbs to make half circles. Apply deep pressure. Glide back down to the ankles.

12

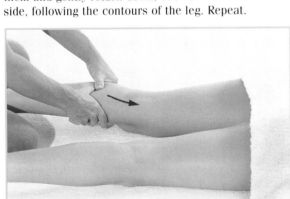

4 Press your thumbs into the centre of the calf muscle, as if you were 'separating' it. Work up to the base of the knee. Repeat.

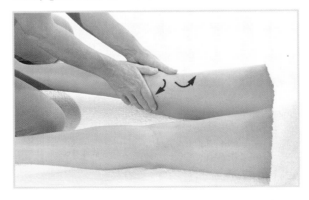

5 Very gently massage the back of the knee, making small circles with your thumbs over the whole of the area.

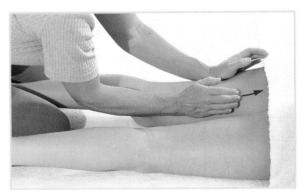

6 Starting just above the knee and working up the whole of the thigh, use the heels of your hands alternately in broad deep, upward strokes.

Move your position to outside the left knee, facing in.

Sinus pain, colds and sore throats

Sinusitis is an inflammation of the nasal sinuses accompanying upper respiratory infection. The sinuses affected are behind the bridge of the nose and in the upper nose, above the eyes and inside each cheekbone. Acute sinusitis is often caused by colds and infections. Symptoms include pain over the forehead and cheekbones, headache, earache, toothache and facial pain.

With colds it is best to allow the mucus to flow without using decongestants, as it is the body's way of ridding itself of the virus.

Sore throats are caused by viral and bacterial infections, usually as an extension of the common cold, although they sometimes result from allergies. Plenty of vitamin C and hot liquids are beneficial for any type of sore throat. If you have a throat infection avoid vigorous massage.

As colds are highly infectious it is best to work on yourself. Give yourself a face and head massage (pages 47–49) followed by a hand massage (page 54).

Use any of the following oils: cardamom, cedarwood, cinnamon, clove, eucalyptus, lavender or tea tree.

During your massage, apply pressure for 3–7 seconds to the points shown below.

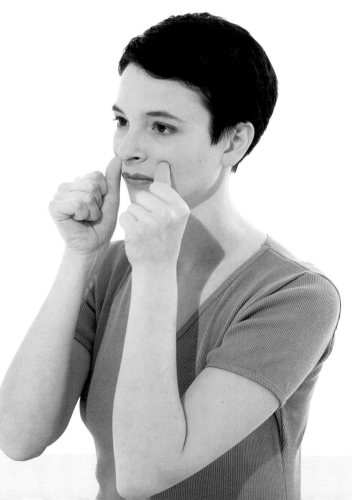

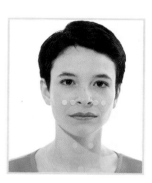

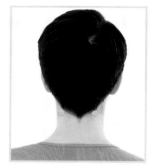

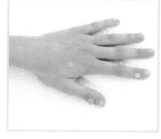

- *Point 1:* Either side of the nose.
- *Point 2:* Under the cheek bones in line with the pupils
- *Point 3:* At base of throat.
- *Point 4:* Level with the top of Adam's apple on the side of the sterno-cleidomastoid muscle.

- *Point 5:* Two points under the occipital ridge midway between the spine and mastoid process.

- *Point 6:* Midway between the first and second metacarpals in the web.
- *Point 7:* Below the nail on the index finger, thumb side.
- *Point 8:* Below the nail on the thumb, farthest side from the fingers.
- *Point 9:* Below the nail on the outer side of the fourth finger.

67

Back of the legs

7 Starting at the top of the outer thigh, use both hands to knead the whole thigh down to the knee. Continue up the middle of the thigh back to the top, then work down the inside.

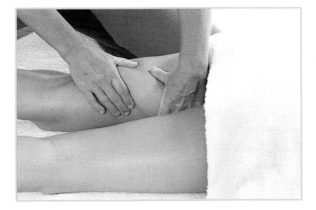

8 Now knead down the inside of the calf, then up the centre to the knee and down the outside edge.

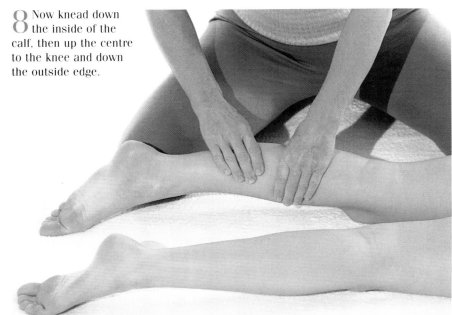

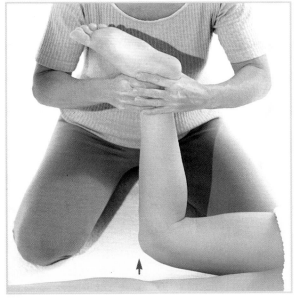

9 Now lift the lower leg so that it forms a right angle to the knee. Use both hands to raise the leg so that the knee is raised slightly off the ground; this will loosen the leg. Return the knee gently to the ground.

13

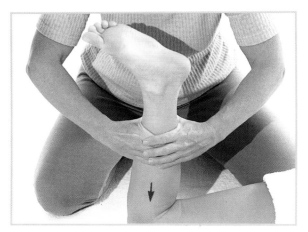

10 With open thumbs and straight fingers, clasp your hands around the ankle and push them down to the knee, squeezing tightly as you do so. Support the leg to prevent it from falling back. Repeat this movement and lower the leg.

Headaches

Stress, tension, anxiety and constipation are some of the various causes of headaches. Tense muscles in the back, shoulders and neck may restrict blood flow to the brain, causing pain. Migraines may begin above one eye or at the back of the head and are sometimes related to food allergy.

But no matter what its cause, massage can help to relieve any type of headache. The type of massage and the pressure points used, however, vary according to the intensity and region of pain.

Ask a friend to massage your headache away – start with the neck and shoulder massage illustrated on pages 34–35.

If you are on your own, however, then do the self massage shown on pages 49–50. Use any of these essential oils in your carrier oil: lavender, rosemary, marjoram, thyme or peppermint.

When you feel relaxed and your muscles are warm then, depending on what type of headache you have, apply pressure to the points pictured below (see chart, right). Usually if you are working on the right point for your pain, it will feel quite tender. Pressure should be applied for 3–7 seconds, using your thumb or your index and middle fingers, and should be as firm as is comfortable for you.

To finish off, massage your feet, working on the big toes (which represent the head in reflexology) as well as under your other toes. Then sit quietly and relax.

> *Frontal headache:* Press points 1 and 2
> *Side headache:* Press point 3
> *Headache in the back of head:*
> Press point 4
> *Migraine:* Press points 5, 8 and 9
> *All headaches:* Press points 6 and 7
> **Avoid pressing points 5 and 7 if you are pregnant.**

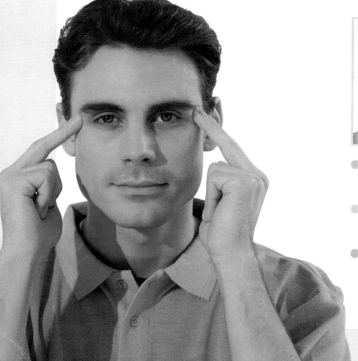

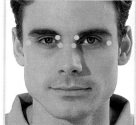

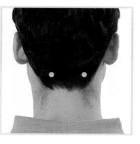

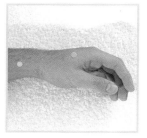

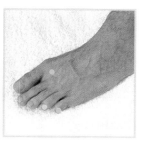

- *Point 1:* Just above and slightly central from the inner corners of the eyes.
- *Point 2:* Just above the previous points, press upwards.
- *Point 3:* In the depression just outside the corner of the eyes.

- *Point 4:* At the central base of the skull just under the ridge. If working on a partner, cradle the head in both hands while applying pressure. Turn the head slightly to one side, then change sides.

- *Point 5:* Press inwards to the centre of the bone between the web.
- *Point 6:* Approximately one and a half thumb widths below the inner wrist crease under the thumb.

- *Point 7:* Just outside the bottom corner of the nail on the little toe.
- *Point 8:* Just outside the bottom corner of the nail on the fourth toe.
- *Point 9:* About one and a half thumb widths in from the web between the big and second toe.

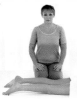

Back of the legs

11 Lift the lower leg again with your right hand. Clasp the ankle with both hands and lift it slightly, wiggling the leg gently to prepare it for the following stretch. Lower the knee.

12 Now place your left hand on the lower back, while your right hand gently pushes the foot towards the buttock. Do not force this movement. Your left hand on the lower back will be feeling for any tension, which indicates when you should stop. Return the foot to above the knee.

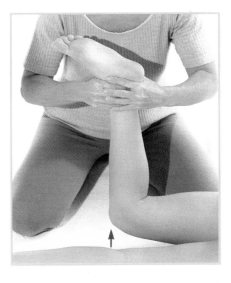

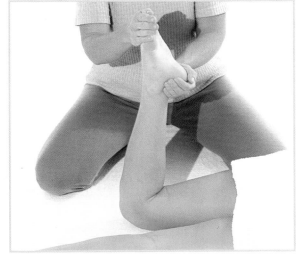

13 Support the heel of your partner's foot in your left hand and push against the top of the foot with your right palm. Stretch the foot so that the toes are pointing.

14

14 Keeping your left hand on the heel, bring your right palm onto the sole of the foot. Gently stretch it down. Return the leg to the ground.

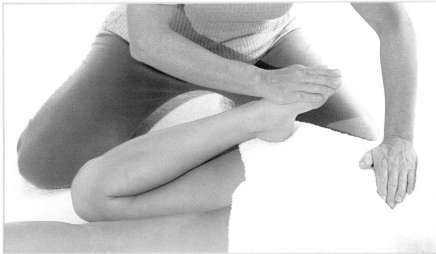

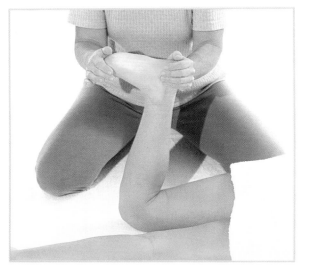

Stress, anxiety and insomnia

Many people suffer from stress as a result of exhausting schedules and other aspects of modern life. Stress is a major contributing factor to conditions such as high blood pressure and heart disease, and lowers immunity to many types of disease. It can also lead to problems such as anxiety and insomnia.

Massage is the natural way to relax and rebalance your body, enabling you to regain both physical and mental health. If you are massaging someone specifically for insomnia, it should be done in the place where the person will be sleeping so that he or she can drop off during or immediately after the massage. If you are giving a massage to a partner follow the complete partnered massage on pages 2–39, omitting the stimulating percussion strokes. If you are massaging yourself follow the self massage routine on pages 47–59, again omitting the percussion strokes.

For stress, use essential oils such as geranium and jasmine, and for anxiety and insomnia use lavender – sprinkle a few drops on your pillow too.

Press into the following points for 3–7 seconds during the course of your massage or press into them whenever necessary.

Stress: Press points 2 and 5
Anxiety and insomnia: Press points 1, 3, 4 and 6

Avoid pressing point 6 if you are pregnant.

65

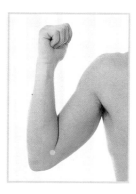

● *Point 1*: At the end of the internal elbow crease, when the arm is bent.

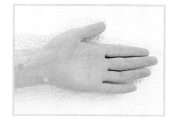

● *Point 2*: On the inside of the wrist, between the two tendons, approximately two thumb widths from the wrist crease.
● *Point 3*: Just below the small bone at the wrist crease on the little finger side.

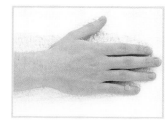

● *Point 4*: On the inside of the little finger just below the nail.

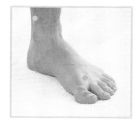

● *Point 5*: About one and a half thumb widths in from the web, between the big and second toe.
● *Point 6*: Four finger widths above the inner ankle – press in at the edge of the bone.

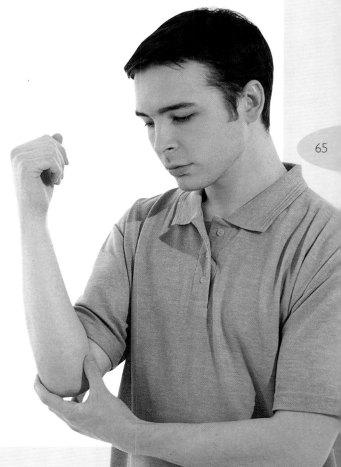

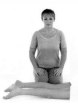

Back of the legs

Avoid these strokes
on the back of the knees
or over bony areas

Adjust your position as
you work, moving up
or down if necessary

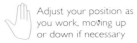

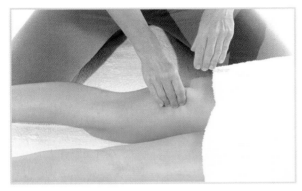

15 Starting at the calf, pluck lumps of flesh between your fingers and thumbs. Work up to the inner thigh, round the outside and back to the calf.

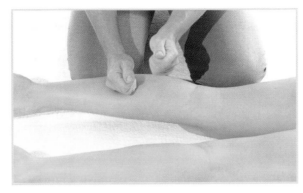

16 Use the sides of loosely clenched fists to pummel against the fleshy parts of the calf and on the inner and outer thigh.

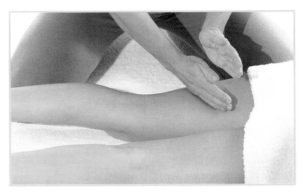

17 Loosen your fingers and use the sides of your hands to create a 'karate chop' or hacking movement over the calf and the whole of the thigh.

15

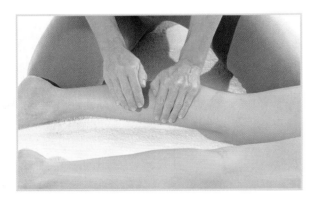

18 Create a cup shape with your palms. Drum your hands against the skin, starting at the calf, then work along the inner thigh.

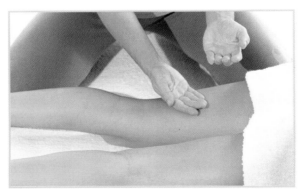

19 Relax your hands and slap the backs lightly against the skin over the fleshy parts of the calf and the whole of the thigh.

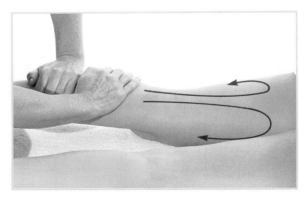

20 Move back down to the foot and do a continuous long stroke up to the thigh, then glide lightly down to the ankle to finish.

Move to the right leg. ◁◁ Repeat steps 1–20. Move back to your partner's left side.

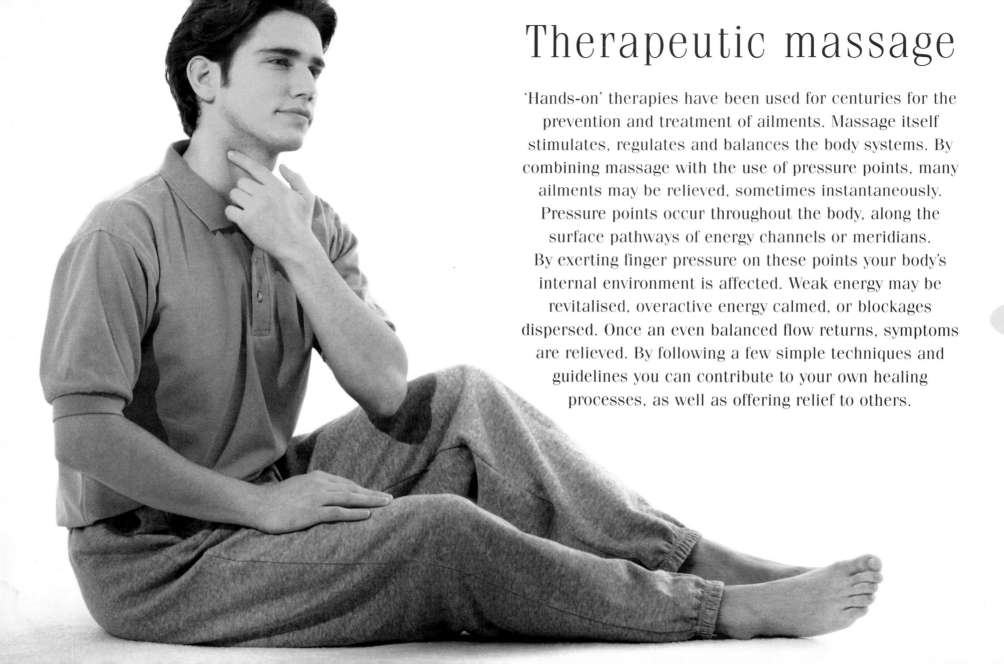

Therapeutic massage

'Hands-on' therapies have been used for centuries for the prevention and treatment of ailments. Massage itself stimulates, regulates and balances the body systems. By combining massage with the use of pressure points, many ailments may be relieved, sometimes instantaneously. Pressure points occur throughout the body, along the surface pathways of energy channels or meridians. By exerting finger pressure on these points your body's internal environment is affected. Weak energy may be revitalised, overactive energy calmed, or blockages dispersed. Once an even balanced flow returns, symptoms are relieved. By following a few simple techniques and guidelines you can contribute to your own healing processes, as well as offering relief to others.

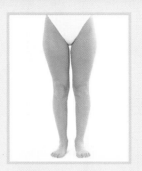

FRONT OF THE LEGS

Compared to the back of the leg, the front is harder and bonier, especially the knee and lower leg, so slightly different techniques are employed within the massage. Deep pressure is only applied on the quadriceps muscles.

Always use stronger pressure working up the leg to improve the circulation and lymphatic drainage.

The inner thigh is included in a front leg massage as it is easily accessed. It may however be ticklish or uncomfortable for some people, so gauge your partner's reaction.

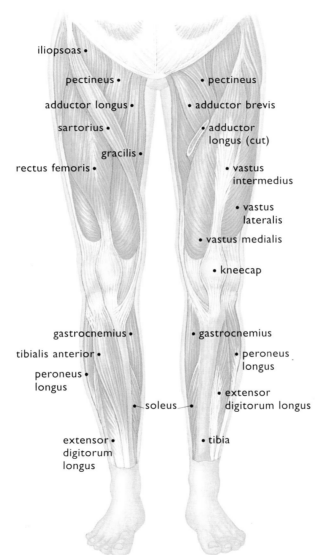

iliopsoas •
pectineus •
adductor longus •
sartorius •
gracilis •
rectus femoris •

• pectineus
• adductor brevis
• adductor longus (cut)
• vastus intermedius
• vastus lateralis
• vastus medialis
• kneecap

gastrocnemius •
tibialis anterior •
peroneus longus •

• gastrocnemius
• peroneus longus
• extensor digitorum longus
• tibia

— soleus •

extensor digitorum longus

◀ **The bones**
The thigh bone (femur) is the largest in the body. The shin bone (tibia) is the stoutest and can be felt close to the surface, while the thinner bone (fibula), to the outside of it, is deeper.

◀ **The quadriceps**
This is a group of four muscles at the front of the thigh (rectus femoris, vastus intermedius, vastus medialis and vastus lateralis) which are often fairly taut and need to be massaged firmly.

◀ **The adductors**
These fleshy muscles of the inner thigh are usually quite relaxed and easy to massage but take care not to work too close to the genitals.

◀ **The kneecap (patella)**
The kneecap is a small bone which should be worked over with very light pressure. Avoid working over it if your partner has had a knee injury.

◀ **The gastrocnemius**
This muscle reaches around the inside of the lower leg from the back of the calf. It is fleshy and can be worked into alongside the bone.

◀ **The tibialis anterior and exterior digitorum longus**
These muscles on the outer side of the shin bone often feel sore when touched.

Note: Superficial muscles are shown on the left leg and deep muscles on the right leg.

16

Self energy quick fix

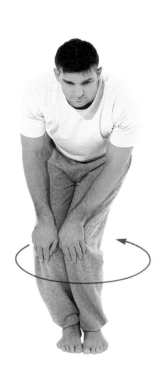

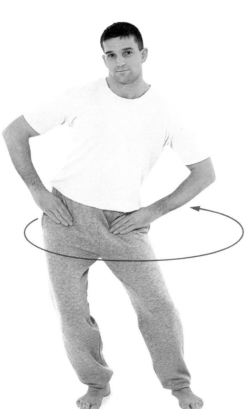

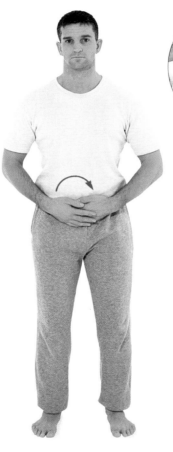

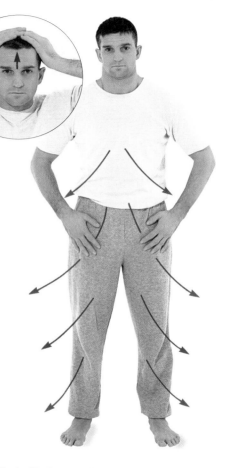

18 Stand with your feet together. Bend your knees and place your hands on top of them. Rotate your knees in a semicircle, straightening your legs as you bring your weight backwards. Repeat, then rotate twice in the opposite direction.

19 Place your hands on your hips and move your feet apart. Bend your knees and slowly rotate your hips in a complete circle. Relax into each position and feel yourself stretching the front of your thighs, hips and lower back. Repeat in the opposite direction.

20 Stand straight with your knees slightly bent. Place one hand just below your navel, with the other on top. Move them around slowly in a large clockwise circle. Repeat this a few times in the same direction then rest your hands in their original position.

21 Shake your hands, then stroke them up over your forehead and the top of your head, down to your neck and across your face. Work down your arms, hands, chest and abdomen, back and buttocks, then legs and feet, as if brushing dust off your clothes.

63

Front of the legs

  Use very light pressure over the kneecap

 If your partner is cold, cover the leg that you are not working on

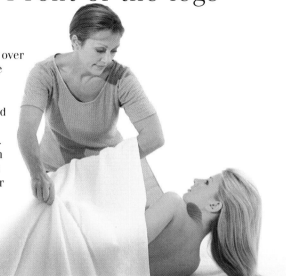

1 Ask your partner to turn over onto her back and as she does so, adjust the towels: scoop your left hand underneath the top towel and grasp the bottom towel at waist level on your nearside. With your right hand, stretch across and take hold of both towels on the outside at your partner's waist level. As she turns, lift the towels slightly. When she is lying flat, straighten the towels.

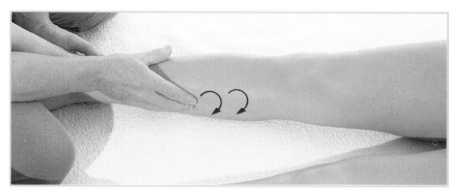

3 Starting at the ankle, use your right hand with fingers close together to make large circle shapes along the inner side of the lower leg up to the knee. Glide back to the ankle. Using your left hand repeat the circular movements on the outer side of the leg. Glide back to the ankle.

17

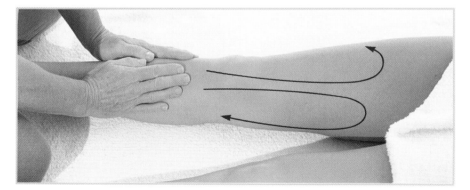

2 Move down opposite the left foot with your knees on either side of your partner's calf. Place your hands just above the ankles with your fingers pointing upwards. With one continuous stroke, glide up to the top of the thigh and back down the sides, following the contours of the leg. Repeat to spread the oil evenly.

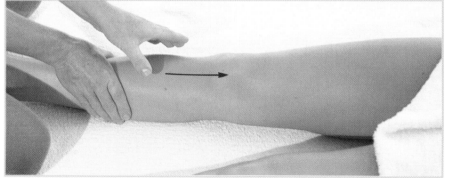

4 Pull your thumbs back making a V-shape (the 'dragon's mouth' position). Place your hands over the shin bone at the base of the leg. Use alternating hands to squeeze slowly up to the base of the knee.

Self energy quick fix

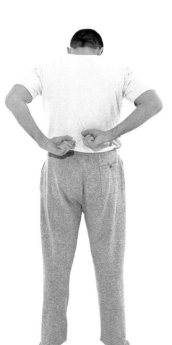

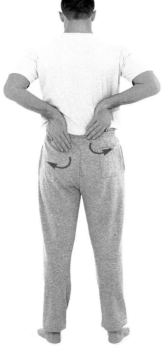

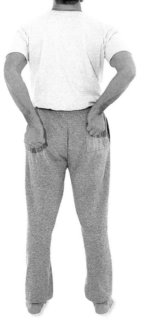

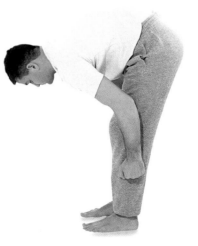

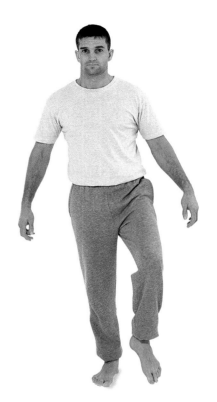

13 Bend forwards slightly and bring your hands up as far as you can comfortably behind your back. Beat down on either side of your spine.

14 Stand up straight and rub your lower back over the kidney area. Continue rubbing until you feel warmth penetrating from your hands. Then rub out towards your hips.

15 Still standing straight, beat both buttocks with loose fists. Alternatively, twist slightly to one side and beat one side at a time.

16 Bend forwards. Using a rhythmic beat and working on both sides of your legs together, work down the insides and down the front. Beat the front of your feet. Return up the back of your legs working on to the buttocks.

17 Stand up straight again and shake each foot and leg several times to loosen them and relieve any tension.

Front of the legs

Use very light pressure over the kneecap

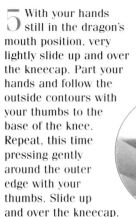

5 With your hands still in the dragon's mouth position, very lightly slide up and over the kneecap. Part your hands and follow the outside contours with your thumbs to the base of the knee. Repeat, this time pressing gently around the outer edge with your thumbs. Slide up and over the kneecap.

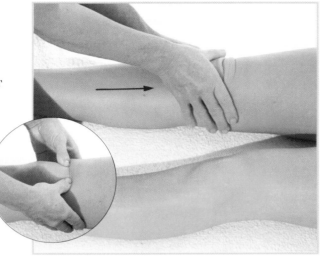

6 With open palms, make upward circular movements over the thigh, pushing with your thumbs as you do so. Work over the top and both sides of the thigh, going up to the hips with the outer hand. Glide back lightly to the side of the knee.

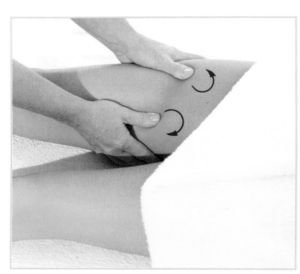

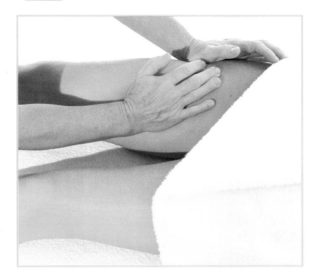

7 Starting just above the knee, use the heels of both hands alternately to push the flesh upwards. Cover the whole of the thigh and work up to the hip.

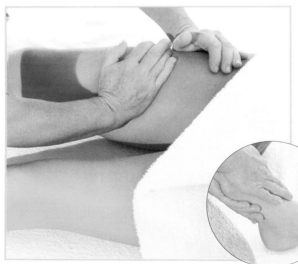

8 Pressing with the outer edge of the palm, make alternating circles from just above the knee to the top of the thigh, pushing into the flesh. With both hands, glide back down the sides of the leg to the ankle and as you reach the foot, lightly press it between your hands and slide your hands over the toes.

18

Self energy quick fix

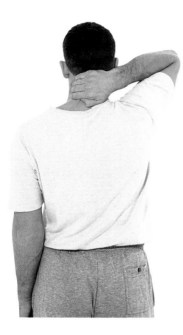

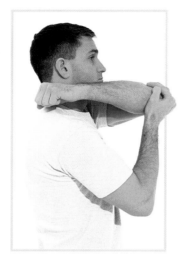

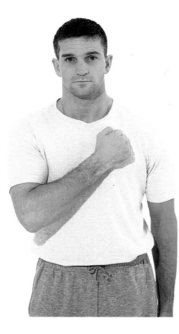

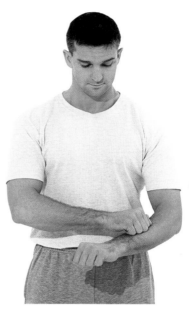

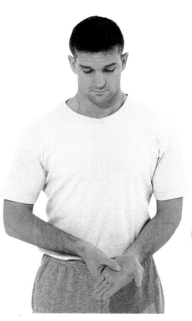

9 Make a loose fist with your right hand. Bring it up to your shoulder, supporting the elbow with your other hand. Bounce the fist along the top and back of your shoulder. Change hands and repeat on the other side.

8 Using one hand, grasp the back of your neck. Squeeze the muscles between your fingers and the heel of your hand working from the base to the top. Change hands and repeat.

10 Form a loose fist with one hand and beat lightly over the opposite chest. Change hands and repeat on the other side. Now use both hands to beat the chest. If you are in an appropriate place, take a deep breath and sing 'ahh' on the outbreath, as you beat.

11 Hold one arm out slightly to the side. Beat down the inside to your hand and beat your palm. Turn your hand over and beat the back of the hand, then up the other side of the arm to the shoulder. If any areas feel tender, which you will probably find on the forearm, beat them for an extra few seconds. Repeat on the other arm.

12 Massage your left palm with your right thumb. One by one, squeeze and pull your fingers and thumb. Repeat on the other hand. Shake both hands and arms.

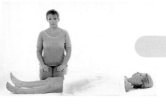

Front of the legs

Do not use these strokes on the knees or bony areas

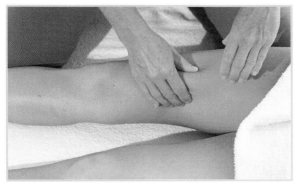

9 Starting at the thigh, pluck and pinch lumps of flesh between your fingers and thumbs. Work down to the calf.

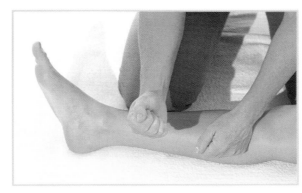

10 With loosely clenched fists, use the sides of your hands to pummel against the inner thigh and calf.

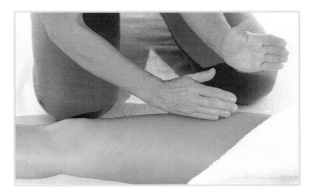

11 With loose fingers, use the sides of your hands to 'karate chop' or hack the flesh. Work on the whole of the thigh, including the area at the side just below the hip.

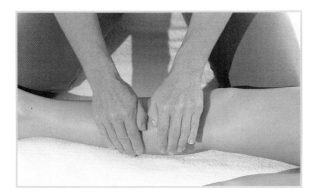

19

12 Cup your hands, keeping fingers together. Drum against the flesh, working along the inner thigh and calf.

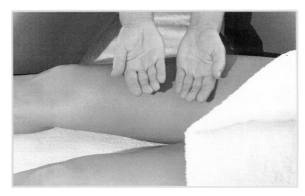

13 Relax your hands and slap the backs lightly against the skin. Use this technique over the whole of the thigh and inner calf.

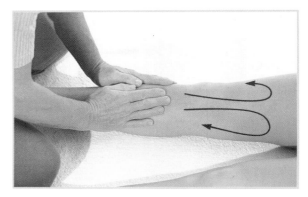

14 Move back down to the foot and finish the leg massage with a continuous long stroke from the ankle to the thigh, gliding back down again. Press the foot between your hands and slide your hands off the toes.

Move to the right leg. ◁◁ Repeat steps 1–14. Then cover both legs with the towel.

Self energy quick fix

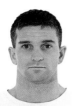

1 Stand with your feet a shoulder width apart and knees slightly bent.

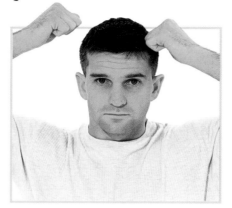

2 Make loose fists and tap from the top of your head down to your neck. Continue tapping in lines moving your hands apart each time. Work from front to back, including the sides.

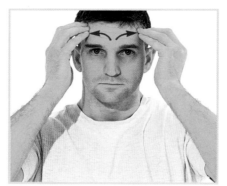

3 Place your fingers between your eyebrows: push up and out gradually covering the whole forehead. Work in lines to cover the forehead.

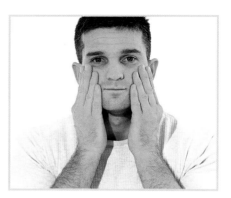

4 Now with flat hands stroke from the bridge of your nose outwards covering the cheeks. Then pinch along your chin and jaw line.

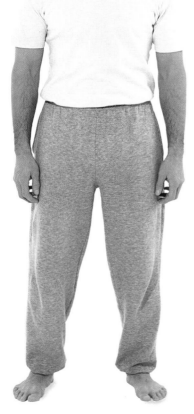

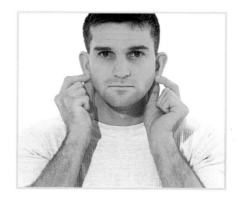

5 Squeeze your ear lobes between your thumbs and fingers. Now massage the bony areas behind your ears in circular movements.

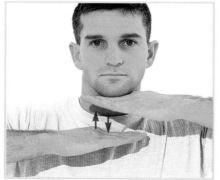

6 Hold one hand horizontally level with your throat and use the other one to bounce off it, patting all around the jawline and under the chin.

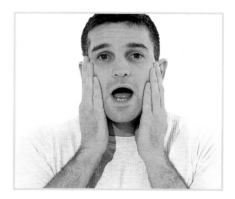

7 Now open your mouth into a wide grin and pat all over your cheeks with flat palms.

60

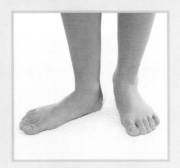

THE FEET

A foot massage is stimulating and revitalising, not only to the feet but to the entire body. Thousands of nerve endings on the soles and a system of reflexes corresponding to the rest of the body, restore balance and assist relaxation, and form the basis of reflexology.

Massaging between the tendons on the top of the foot is beneficial for the circulation and lymphatic drainage but can feel quite tender for some people.

The massage techniques on the following pages will relax the feet and keep them flexible, as well as helping your partner's overall well-being.

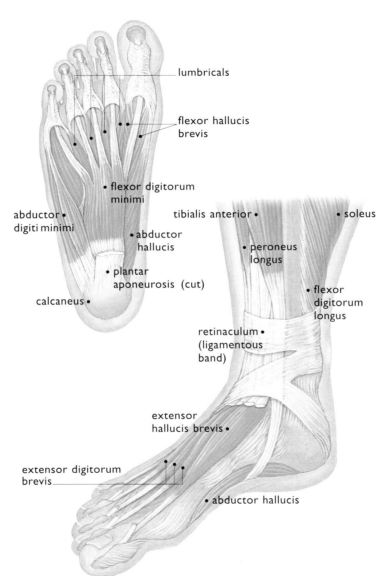

lumbricals

flexor hallucis brevis

• flexor digitorum minimi

abductor• digiti minimi

tibialis anterior •

• soleus

• abductor hallucis

• peroneus longus

• plantar aponeurosis (cut)

calcaneus •

• flexor digitorum longus

retinaculum • (ligamentous band)

extensor hallucis brevis •

extensor digitorum brevis

• abductor hallucis

◄ The arch of the foot
The curve of the arch has reflexes which relate to the spine in reflexology. Using deep pressure here may bring relief for a backache.

◄ The toes
Along the bottom of the toes are reflexes relating to the head, sinuses, eyes, ears and teeth in reflexology. When massaged they bring relief from problems experienced in these areas.

◄ The tarsals and metatarsals
Each foot contains 26 bones: seven bones of the ankle, the tarsals; five of the foot, the metatarsals; and 14 of the toes, the phalanges. Massaging between these bones has a beneficial effect.

◄ The sole
The heel of the foot and balls of the toes (which are covered with tough layers of skin) can take deep pressure, but use slightly less over the middle of the sole, underneath the instep.

20

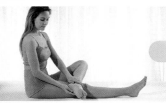

The feet

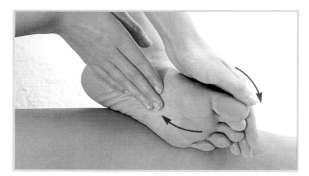

1 Sit on the ground and bring your left foot to rest on your right thigh. Place your right hand on the sole with the left hand on top of the foot. Stroke down with the right hand and up with the left hand over the toes, in a continuous movement.

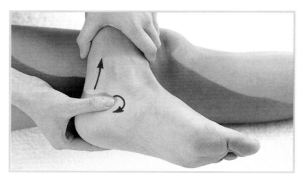

2 Let your foot hang over your thigh. Using your thumb, work on the inner side of the heel, from the instep to the ankle. Use circular movements and static pressure. Then squeeze upwards along the tendon at the back of the ankles.

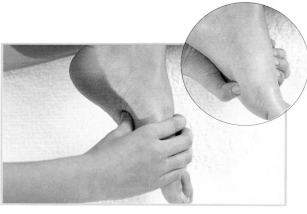

3 With your thumb under your foot, use your index finger to press downwards between the tendons of the big and second toe. Work down the next two grooves, then bring your hand underneath to work on the outer side with your index and middle fingers.

59

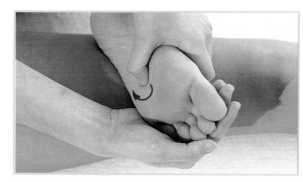

4 Draw your foot up to rest across your thigh and massage the sole with circular movements with your left hand or both hands. Using your thumb, press in lines towards each toe using small but deep movements.

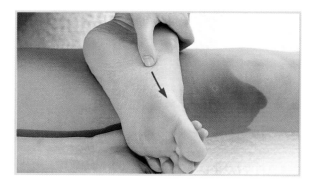

5 With your left hand 'caterpillar walk' the thumb along the side of the instep, to the base of the big toe, following the curve just underneath the bones. Then repeat the movement along the bone itself.

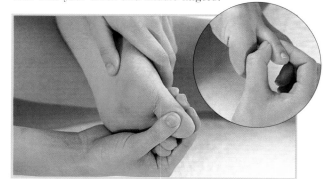

6 One by one press into the underside of each of the toes, from the base to the tip, covering the middle and both sides. Now squeeze and pull with your fingers and thumb, first along the edges, then from the bottom and the top. ◁◁ Repeat step 1.

◁◁ Repeat steps 1–6 on the other foot.

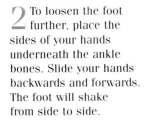

The feet

Ask your partner if he or she has any painful corns before massaging the feet

1 Place a large cushion under your partner's feet and another one under her knees. Then loosely cup your palms around the sides of her right foot. Relax your fingers and move your hands rapidly backwards and forwards. This will relax the foot.

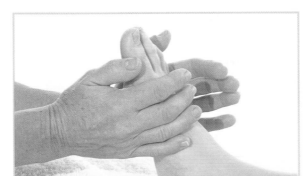

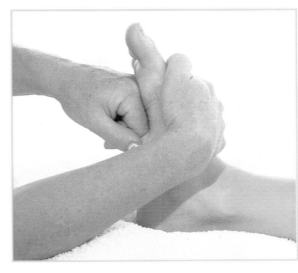

3 Make your left hand into a fist and place it against the ball of the foot. Wrap your right hand over the top of the foot with fingers on the outside. Work the hands alternately, pushing with the left, then squeezing with the right.

21

2 To loosen the foot further, place the sides of your hands underneath the ankle bones. Slide your hands backwards and forwards. The foot will shake from side to side.

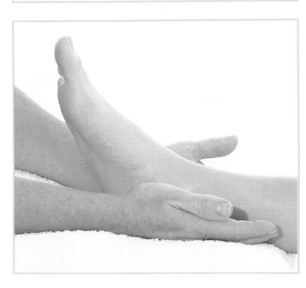

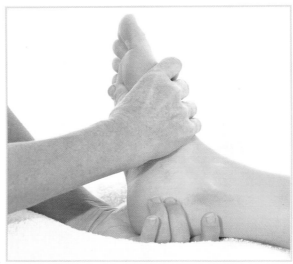

4 Keep your right hand over the top of the foot. Move your left hand down and slip it under the right heel. Gently pull the foot towards you from the heel. Using an oval motion, rotate the foot a few times in each direction.

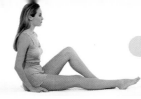

The legs

 Optional

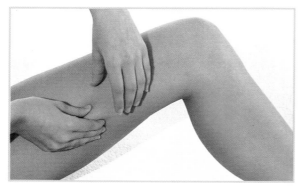

9 Pluck the inner thigh with both hands working up and down the muscles.

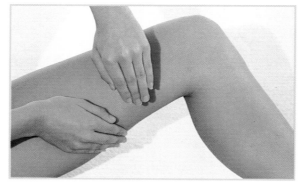

10 Cup your hands as if to scoop water and then drum against the whole of the inner thigh.

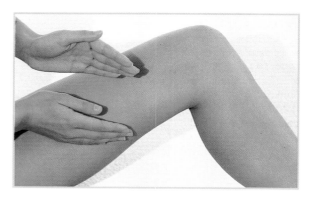

11 With loose fingers, 'karate chop' or 'hack' your inner thigh with the sides of your hands.

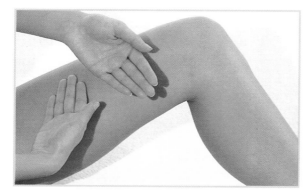

12 Use the back of your hands to slap the inner thigh. Keep the hands relaxed as they bounce off the flesh.

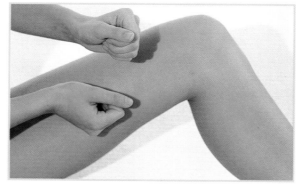

13 Make loose fists and pummel your inner thigh rapidly. Turn your foot in once again.
◁◁ Repeat steps 9–13 on the outer thigh and hip.

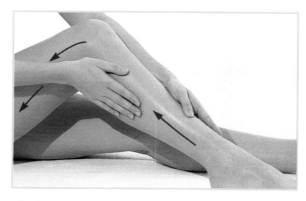

14 Finish by stroking up the whole leg with flat hands. Start at the front of the ankle, stroke up the leg then repeat up the back of the leg.

Turn back to page 56. ◁◁ Repeat steps 1–14 on the other leg.

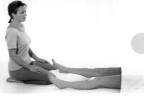

The feet

Use a very small amount of oil if necessary

5 Place your thumbs on top of the foot at the ankle, with your fingers underneath the foot. Push your thumbs apart in an opening movement. Work down to the base of the toes.

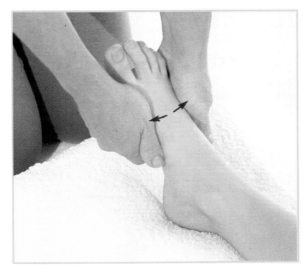

7 Holding the foot in your left hand, press and pinch around the edges of the heel with your right thumb and index finger. Now thumb press across the base of the heel.

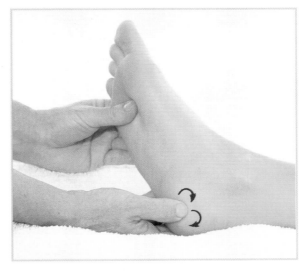

6 Hold the foot in your left hand using your thumb under the ball of the big toe for support. Now with your right thumb massage the right side of the sole with small circular movements, working from the heel to the base of the toes. Work in towards the centre. Change your hands and work from the other side.

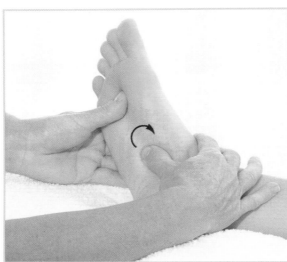

8 Hold the foot with your left hand and cup your right palm under the heel. With your right thumb 'caterpillar walk' from the middle side of the heel to the beginning of the instep. Now bring your fingers over the top of the foot, allowing your thumb to continue 'walking' along the side of the instep, under the curve of the bone, to the big toe.

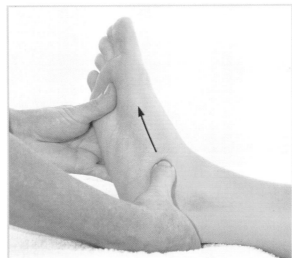

22

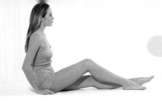

The legs

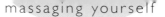

Optional

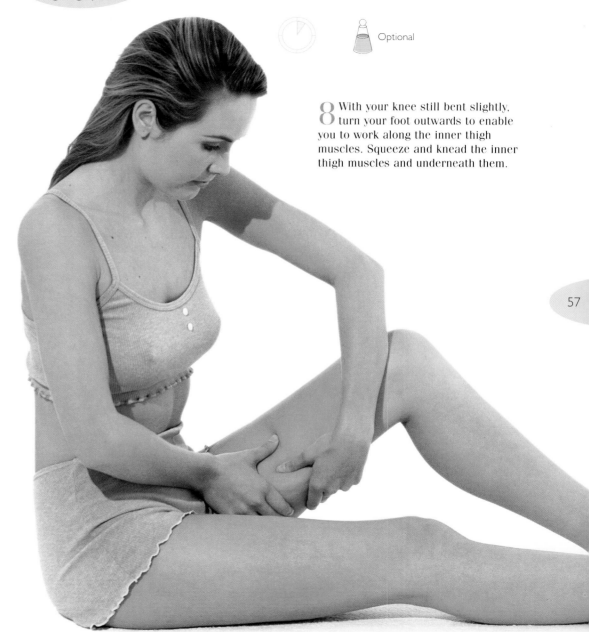

8 With your knee still bent slightly, turn your foot outwards to enable you to work along the inner thigh muscles. Squeeze and knead the inner thigh muscles and underneath them.

57

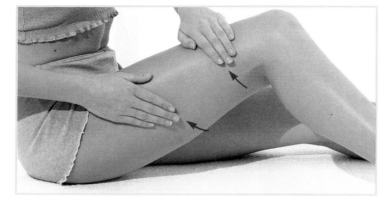

6 Slightly bend the leg that you are working on. Starting at the knee, use both hands to stroke firmly upwards. Cover the whole thigh on top and underneath.

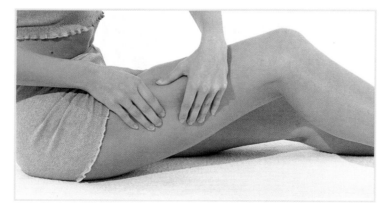

7 Now knead the top of the thigh from the knee out diagonally to the hip. Turn your foot inwards slightly if this makes it easier to knead effectively.

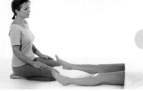

The feet

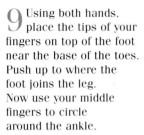

9 Using both hands, place the tips of your fingers on top of the foot near the base of the toes. Push up to where the foot joins the leg. Now use your middle fingers to circle around the ankle.

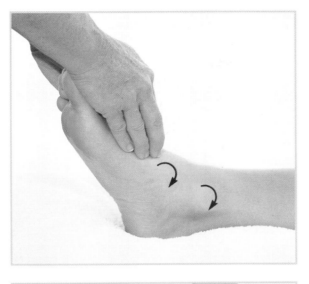

10 Hold the foot with thumbs on top of it and fingers underneath. Starting with the web between the big and second toes, use your thumbs to press down between the tendons. Repeat this movement along each of the grooves.

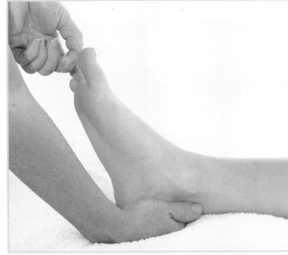

11 Hold the heel of the foot with your right hand. Use your left thumb and index fingers to pull and squeeze the toes. First place your thumb on top of the big toe, index finger underneath, now rub and pull off the end. Using the same movement, work down the sides of the toe. Now work along the other toes using the same technique.

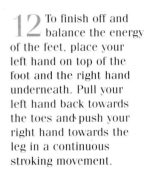

23

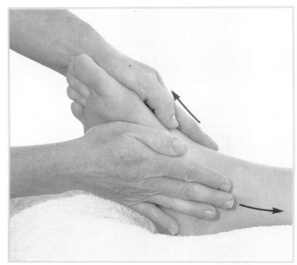

12 To finish off and balance the energy of the feet, place your left hand on top of the foot and the right hand underneath. Pull your left hand back towards the toes and push your right hand towards the leg in a continuous stroking movement.

◁◁ Repeat steps 1–12 on the left foot. Then cover the feet and move to your partner's right side at hip level.

The legs

  Optional

1 Sit up and bend the leg you are going to massage. Keep your foot flat on the ground. Starting at the ankle, firmly stroke up to the knee, first at the front then at the back. Keep hands flat but not rigid.

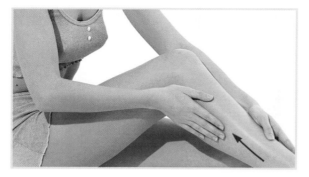

2 Beginning above the Achilles tendon behind your ankle, alternate your hands to squeeze and knead the calf muscles between your fingers and thumbs.

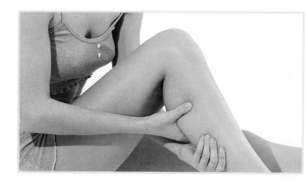

3 Bring your fingers around the front of your leg and push both thumbs into the centre of the calf muscles. Press in and hold for about 7 seconds, moving upwards 1 cm at a time until you reach the knee. Repeat over any tender points.

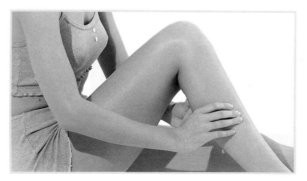

4 Stroke your hands gently over the top of your knee. Bring your elbows out and use your thumbs to press around the kneecap.

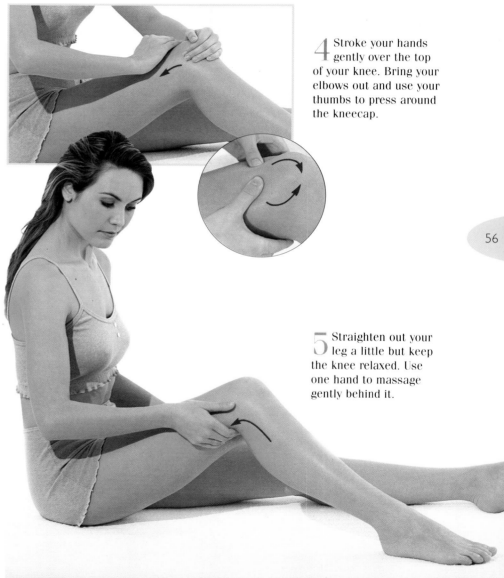

5 Straighten out your leg a little but keep the knee relaxed. Use one hand to massage gently behind it.

56

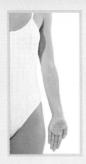

THE HANDS AND ARMS

A hand massage may be given anywhere with no disrobing or preparation necessary and because of the many pressure points on the hands, it produces a relaxing effect throughout the body. It is an excellent way of conveying comfort and caring to people of any age.

The arms sustain a lot of physical strain during the day and often hold enormous amounts of tension, which travels up into the shoulders and neck, causing discomfort.

Massage and passive stretches can help to let go of this tension. Before massaging the arm raise it slightly and wiggle it to help the muscles relax.

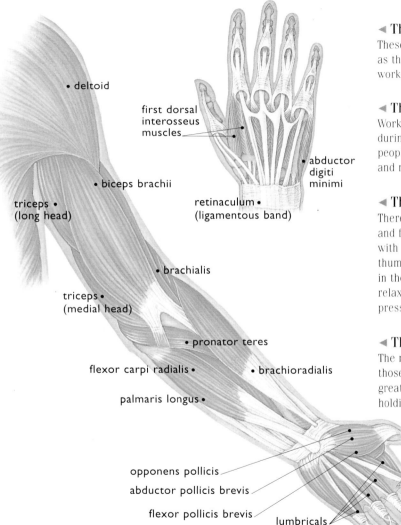

- deltoid
- biceps brachii
- triceps • (long head)
- first dorsal interosseus muscles
- abductor digiti minimi
- retinaculum (ligamentous band)
- brachialis
- triceps (medial head)
- pronator teres
- flexor carpi radialis •
- brachioradialis
- palmaris longus •
- opponens pollicis
- abductor pollicis brevis
- flexor pollicis brevis
- lumbricals

24

◄ The deltoid, biceps and triceps

These muscles in the upper arm as well as the muscles of the forearm can all be worked into deeply to promote relaxation.

◄ The elbow

Work into and around the elbow joint during your massage. Note that some people are sensitive around the elbow and may not like pressure around it.

◄ The carpals and metacarpals

There are eight carpal bones in the wrist and five metacarpal bones in the hand, with 14 phalanges in the fingers and thumbs. Massaging between these bones, in the 'web' of the hand is extremely relaxing and also benefits various pressure points.

◄ The hand muscles

The muscles of the hand, particularly those at the base of the thumb store a great deal of tension from gripping and holding. Deep pressure massage as well as hand stretches will be extremely soothing.

◄ The wrists

Always support the wrists well and use minimum force when massaging and stretching them.

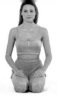

The abdomen

   Optional

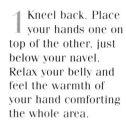

1 Kneel back. Place your hands one on top of the other, just below your navel. Relax your belly and feel the warmth of your hand comforting the whole area.

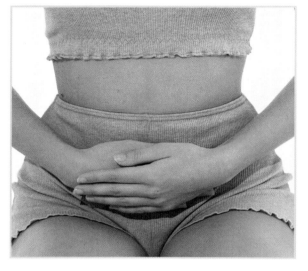

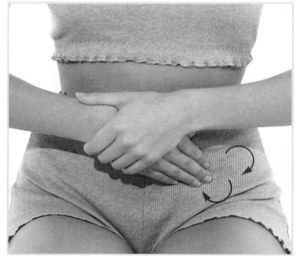

3 Still using a reinforced hand, straighten your fingers and massage around the abdomen in smaller circles.

55

2 Slowly glide your reinforced hand around in a large clockwise circle, three or four times.

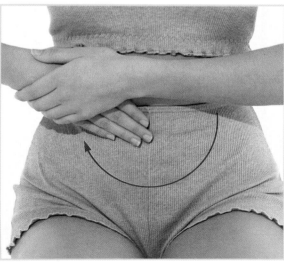

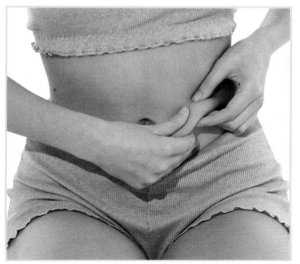

4 Knead and pinch the flesh with your fingers and thumbs, continuing to work in a clockwise direction. Repeat step 1 then bring your hands to rest just below the navel. Close your eyes. Relax and feel the heat from your hands penetrating and soothing your body.

The hands

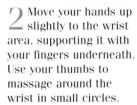

1 Uncover your partner's right arm. Lift the hand and place your fingers under the palm, with the base of your thumbs on the top of the hand. Pull your hands apart, opening and stretching the back of your partner's hand. Now pull your fingers apart underneath to stretch the palm.

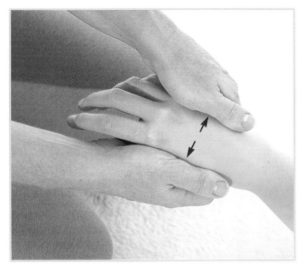

2 Move your hands up slightly to the wrist area, supporting it with your fingers underneath. Use your thumbs to massage around the wrist in small circles.

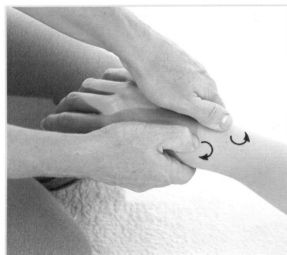

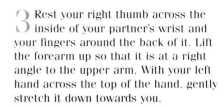

3 Rest your right thumb across the inside of your partner's wrist and your fingers around the back of it. Lift the forearm up so that it is at a right angle to the upper arm. With your left hand across the top of the hand, gently stretch it down towards you.

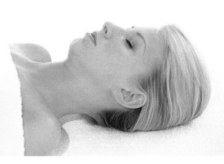

25

4 With your right hand still supporting the wrist, gently stretch your partner's palm and fingers back using your left hand.

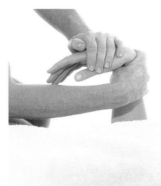

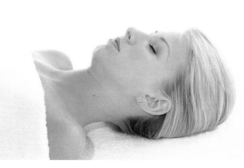

The hands

 Optional

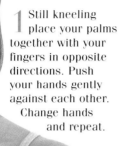

1 Still kneeling place your palms together with your fingers in opposite directions. Push your hands gently against each other. Change hands and repeat.

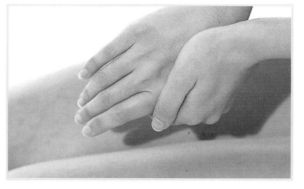

2 Place the heel of one hand over the back of the other, fingers underneath the palm. Squeeze on both sides.

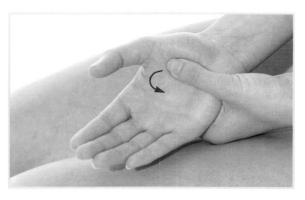

3 Turn one hand to face upwards. Massage around the palm using your thumb in small circular movements. Then apply static pressure. Give particular attention to the large muscle at the base of the thumb.

54

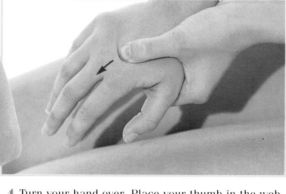

4 Turn your hand over. Place your thumb in the web between the thumb and index finger. Squeeze and press down between the tendons. Repeat a few times then work down the other grooves.

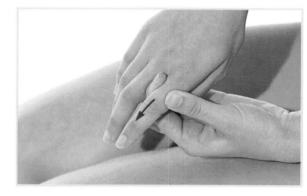

5 Squeeze along each finger and thumb from the base to the tip. First work along the top and then along the sides.

◁◁ Repeat steps 2–5 on the other hand.

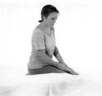

The hands

5 Turn the palm of your partner's hand towards you. Using your thumbs in tiny circular movements, work across the underside of the wrist. Gradually work into the big muscles at the base of the thumb and little finger.

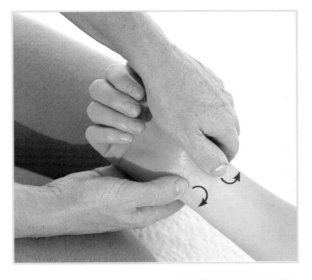

6 Slide your left little finger between your partner's index finger and thumb and your right little finger between your partner's ring and little fingers. Bring the rest of your fingers underneath and your thumbs onto the palm. Stretch the palm open as you pull your thumbs back and push up with your fingers from underneath. Then massage the palm with your thumbs, using small circular movements.

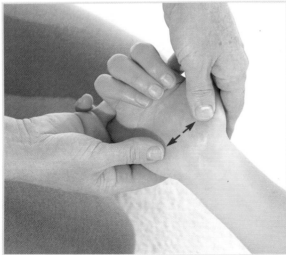

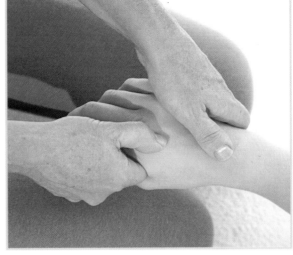

7 Turn the hand over and support the wrist with your left hand. Using your right thumb on top and your index finger underneath, squeeze down between the bones. Work down each of the grooves on the back of the hand, changing your hands if necessary.

26

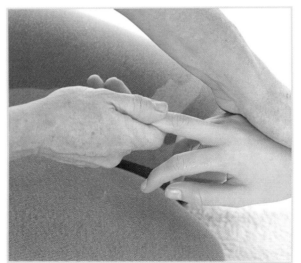

8 Still supporting your partner's hand with your left hand, use your right thumb and index finger to squeeze down the sides of the little finger towards the nail, pulling gently. Now squeeze along the top and bottom and pull off the tip. Work along all of the fingers and the thumb, changing your hands halfway.

Now move slightly up the body to begin massaging the arm.

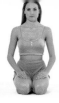

The arms

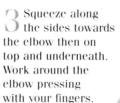 Optional

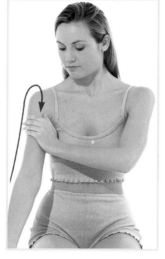

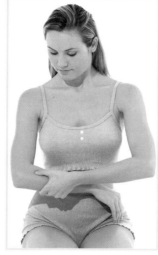

1 Kneel and sit back. Starting at the wrist, firmly stroke up the whole arm, over the back of the shoulder, and lightly down the inner arm. Repeat a couple of times.

2 Bend your arm, as if it was resting in a sling. Massage the inner forearm with your thumb working upwards, then turn your arm over and press into the muscles on top of it.

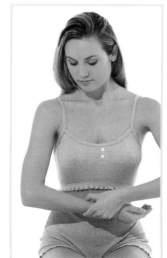

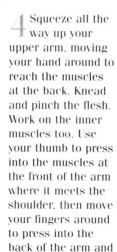

3 Squeeze along the sides towards the elbow then on top and underneath. Work around the elbow pressing with your fingers.

4 Squeeze all the way up your upper arm, moving your hand around to reach the muscles at the back. Knead and pinch the flesh. Work on the inner muscles too. Use your thumb to press into the muscles at the front of the arm where it meets the shoulder, then move your fingers around to press into the back of the arm and shoulder joint.

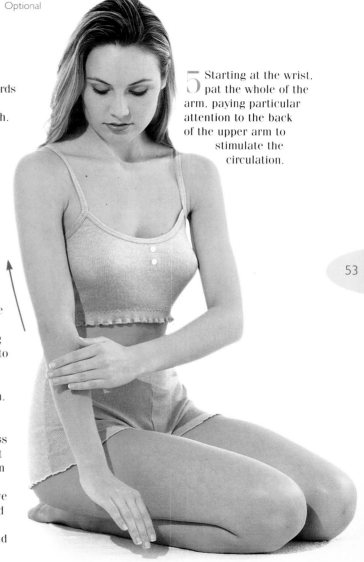

5 Starting at the wrist, pat the whole of the arm, paying particular attention to the back of the upper arm to stimulate the circulation.

53

◁◁ Repeat steps 1–5 on the other arm.

The arms

Always use lighter pressure when you return down the arm toward the hand

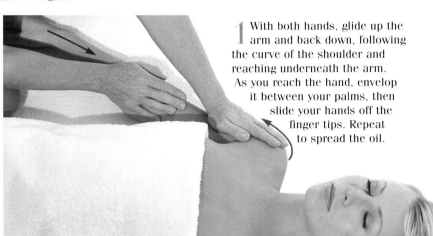

1 With both hands, glide up the arm and back down, following the curve of the shoulder and reaching underneath the arm. As you reach the hand, envelop it between your palms, then slide your hands off the finger tips. Repeat to spread the oil.

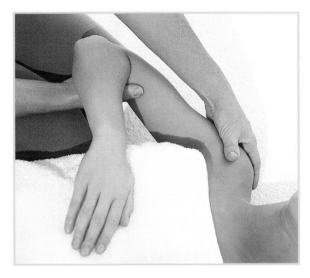

3 Lift your partner's elbow and place her hand on her abdomen. Support the elbow with your right hand. With your left hand, massage the upper arm using circular movements, then squeeze the flesh between fingers and thumb. Work around the shoulder drawing your flat hand underneath. Work on the arm down to the elbow.

27

2 Hold your partner's hand so that the forearm is slightly raised. Use your right thumb in a circular movement to work from the wrist upwards. Switch your hands as you work covering all sides. Then move slightly up the body to the elbow.

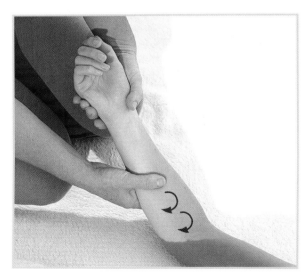

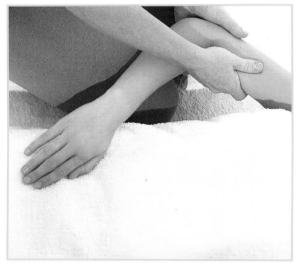

4 Now switch hands and support the elbow with your left hand, bringing it out away from the body slightly. With your right hand, squeeze the flesh on the inside of the upper arm between your thumb and fingers.

Move slightly higher up the body and face inwards.

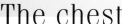

The chest

  Optional

1 Kneel and sit back. Place the three middle fingers of your right hand at the base of your throat. Working towards the opposite shoulder, massage in small circles underneath the collar bone. Bring your hand back to the centre, this time at a slightly lower position and work outwards covering the whole of the upper chest.

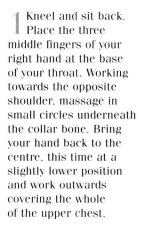

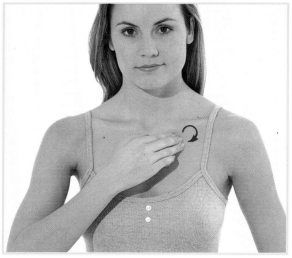

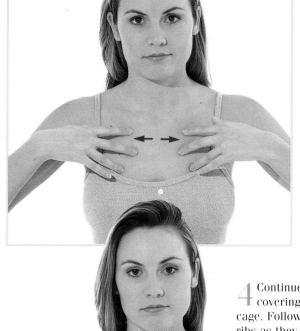

3 Women should only work above and below the breast tissue, but men can use this technique over the whole chest area. Open the middle fingers of both hands and place them vertically in the centre of your upper chest. Draw them apart about 1 cm, to place them in the grooves between the ribs and press inwards for a few seconds. Work out towards the sides.

52

2 Rest the back of your left hand on your left thigh. Now put the fingers of your right hand under your left armpit with your thumb on the pectoral muscle at the top of the breast area. Squeeze into this muscle working towards the centre of your chest. ◁◁ Repeat steps 1 and 2 on the right side.

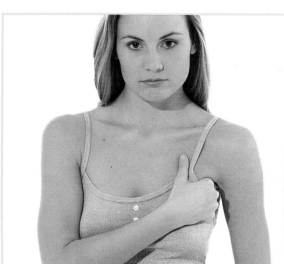

4 Continue with this technique covering the whole of the rib cage. Follow the contours of the ribs as they curve up the sides.

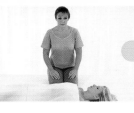

The arms

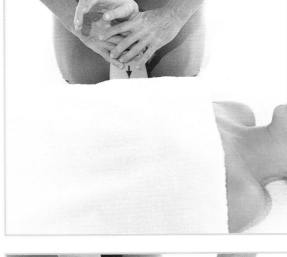

5 Lift your partner's hand so that the forearm is at a right angle. Clasp the fingers and thumbs of both your hands firmly around the wrist. Now squeeze down to the elbow.

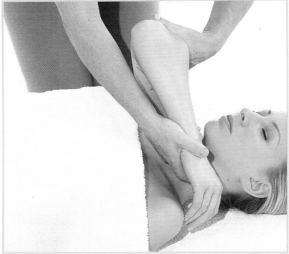

6 Bring your right hand up to the wrist, leaving your left fingers and thumb around the base of the forearm near the elbow. As you do the next step, move upwards to shoulder level. Lift the elbow into a right angle above the shoulder, taking your partner's hand to rest on the opposite side of her neck.

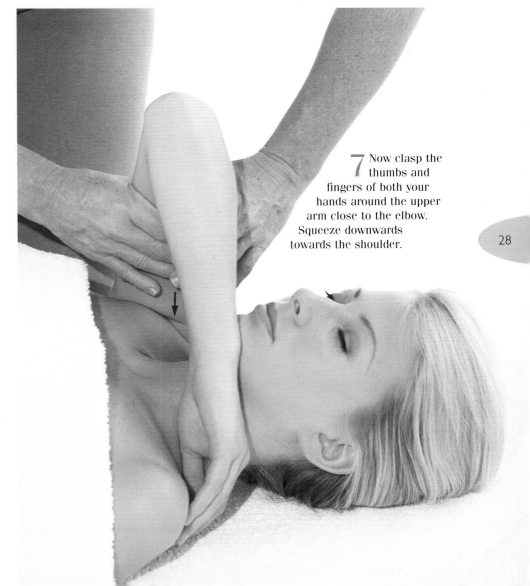

7 Now clasp the thumbs and fingers of both your hands around the upper arm close to the elbow. Squeeze downwards towards the shoulder.

28

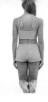

The back

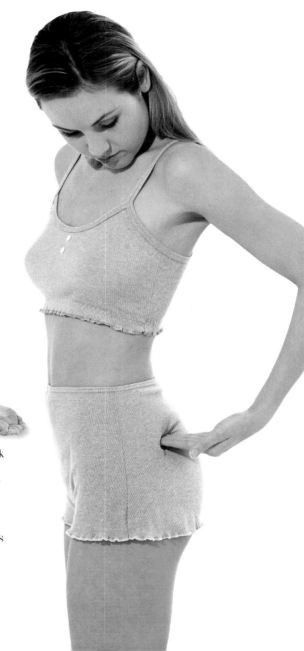

Optional

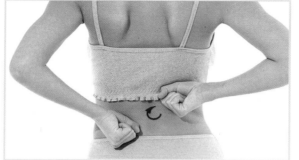

1 Kneel up. Make loose fists and bring both hands behind your back, as high as you can on either side of the spine. Rub in alternating circles up and down your back, covering the sides and lower back as well.

2 Place your thumbs on your waist, with your fingers flat against your back. Squeeze as much flesh in your hands as you can, working upwards. Now bring your fingers forwards and pinch the flesh along the sides of your rib cage.

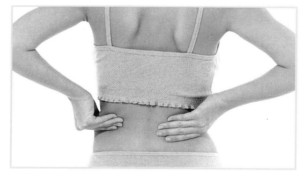

3 Place your hands on your waist with your thumbs either side of your spine. Press in for about 10 seconds. Gradually work downwards. Press into your sacrum and then work outwards covering your lower back.

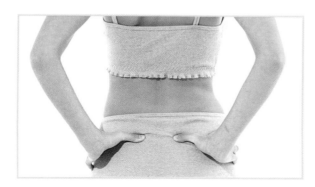

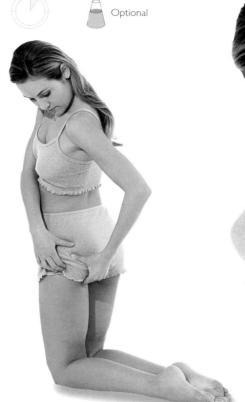

4 Twist your body to enable both hands to work on one buttock at a time. Grab and squeeze handfuls of flesh from the hip area to the lower back, then over the whole cheek.

5 Straighten the middle three fingers of your hand and press into the buttock in small circles. ◁◁ Repeat steps 4 and 5 on the other side of your buttocks.

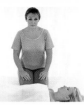

The arms

8 Bring your right knee up. Slide the crook of your left elbow under your partner's elbow. Place your right hand over her forearm and press down to anchor it. Now raise your body, lifting your partner's shoulder off the floor and stretch it gently.

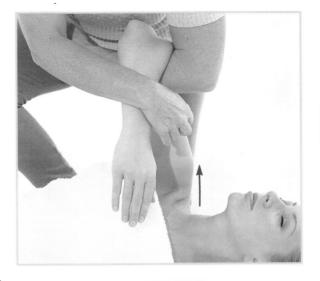

10 Grasp your partner's right wrist in your left hand. Stretch her arm straight up over her head. Slide your other hand down the side of her rib cage towards the hip.

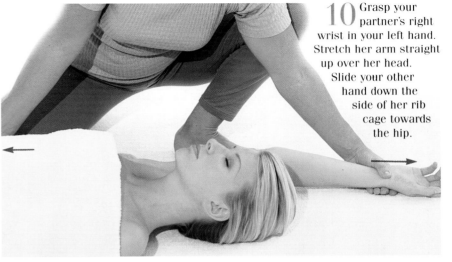

29

9 Place your partner's hand on her opposite shoulder. Kneel down and place the heel of your left hand on top of her right shoulder. Place the heel of your right hand against her elbow. Now at the same time press down on the shoulder and up at the elbow.

11 Lower your partner's arm. Starting at the wrist, use a long stroke to glide up and over the shoulder and all the way back down. Then press the hand between your palms and slide your hand off the fingers. Cover your partner's arm and hand. Move to your partner's left side. ◁◁ Repeat pages 25–29 on the left hand and arm.

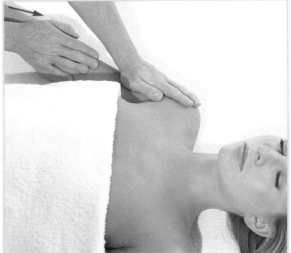

Then move to your partner's right side at waist level, facing in.

The neck and shoulders

 Optional

1 Kneel and sit back on your heels. Relax your shoulders and roll your head around in half circles to each side. Then place one hand over the top of your head. Pull it down towards your shoulder. Change the angle a few times. For a stronger stretch, push the palm of your other hand down towards the ground. Repeat on the other side.

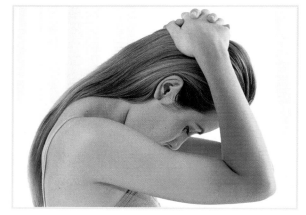

2 Clasp your hands behind your head, bringing your elbows forwards. Now pull your chin down towards your chest and stay in this position for about one minute. This movement stretches the back of the neck and is a very effective technique for dealing with tension and headaches.

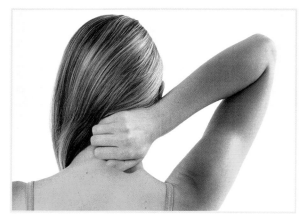

3 With one hand, grasp the back of your neck. Working from the base to the top and back again, squeeze the muscles between your fingers and the heel of your hand. Now repeat this movement with your other hand.

50

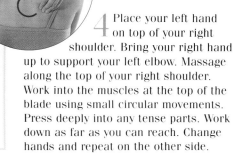

4 Place your left hand on top of your right shoulder. Bring your right hand up to support your left elbow. Massage along the top of your right shoulder. Work into the muscles at the top of the blade using small circular movements. Press deeply into any tense parts. Work down as far as you can reach. Change hands and repeat on the other side.

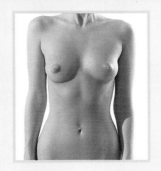

THE ABDOMEN AND CHEST

Always treat the front of the body with extra sensitivity when massaging it as it is the most vulnerable area of the body. The stomach area can also be very ticklish and uncomfortable for some people. Your partner should not eat for at least two hours before being massaged in this area.

When massaging the chest area always avoid the breast tissue in women. Massage above and below the breasts. For men, you can work over the whole chest.

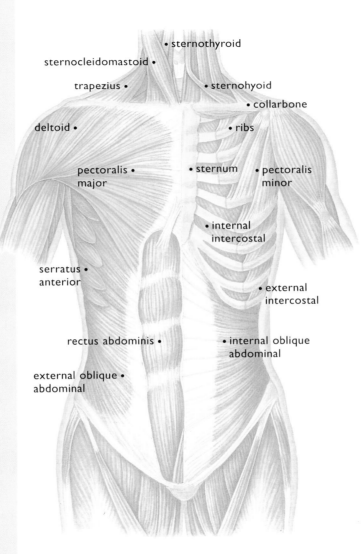

- sternothyroid
- sternocleidomastoid
- trapezius
- sternohyoid
- collarbone
- deltoid
- ribs
- pectoralis major
- sternum
- pectoralis minor
- internal intercostal
- serratus anterior
- external intercostal
- rectus abdominis
- internal oblique abdominal
- external oblique abdominal

◄ **The pectoral muscles**
These pectoralis major and minor are usually more developed in men than in women. They can be kneaded with deep pressure.

◄ **The rib cage**
The chest and rib cage protect and contain vital organs such as the heart and lungs. Applying pressure to certain points may relieve chest ailments (see page 71).

◄ **The intercostal muscles**
These muscles between the ribs enable your rib cage to expand as you breathe in. Massaging them increases flexibility and can improve your breathing.

◄ **The abdomen**
It is essential to massage the abdomen in a clockwise direction, no matter what techniques you use as this is the direction in which food is passed through the intestines.

Note: The left side of the diagram shows superficial muscles and the right side deep muscles.

30

The head

1 Remain in a comfortable sitting position. Stroke upwards over your forehead using alternate hands. Stroke over the top of your head and down to the nape of your neck, then from the temples around the sides of your head.

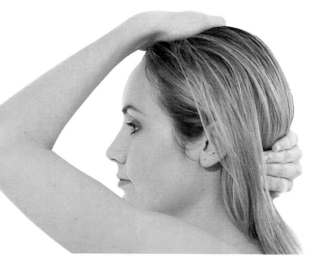

2 Rub all over your scalp with your fingertips as if you are shampooing your hair. Cover the whole of your head, paying particular attention to any sensitive or tense areas.

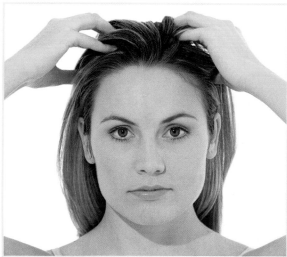

3 Grab handfuls of hair close to the roots and pull them gently to stimulate the hair follicles.

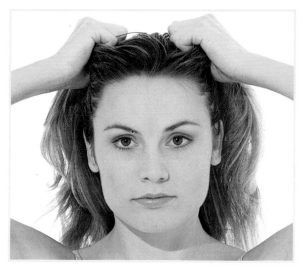

49

4 Press upwards underneath the bony ridge at the base of your skull with your thumbs. Work from behind each ear first and in towards the centre. Roll your head backwards slightly to achieve the best positions. On this area there are several pressure points for the relief of headaches and tension (see page 66).

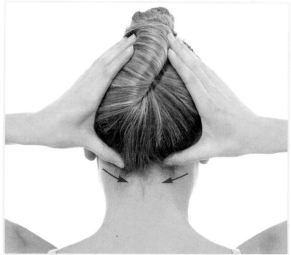

The abdomen

  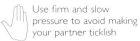

Use firm and slow pressure to avoid making your partner ticklish

1 Fold up the bottom of the top towel to uncover the abdomen. Gently place both your hands on the abdomen and remain still for a few seconds. In a clockwise direction, use the palms of your hands in broad circles around the whole abdomen (the right hand moves behind the left then breaks contact and comes over the left wrist).

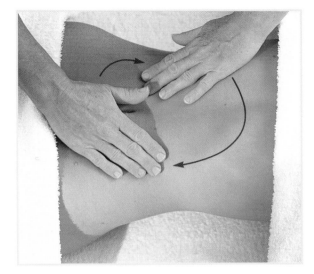

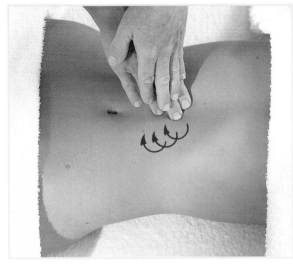

3 Still resting your left hand over your right glide down to approximately 5 cm above the navel. Using slightly deeper pressure and working in a clockwise direction, form small circles with your fingers massaging around the belly.

31

2 Work in a diamond shape: with your left hand on top of the right glide your fingers up between the ribs. From here slide your fingers out over the waist. Pull up, then use the heel of your hand moving down towards the pubic bone. Turn the heel towards you and pull down over the nearside waist. Glide your fingers up between the ribs to the top of the diamond shape.

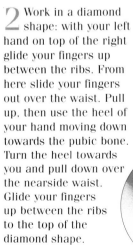

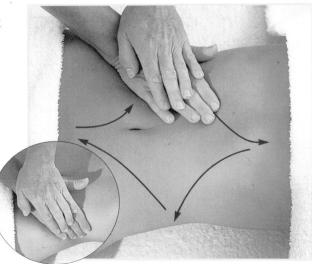

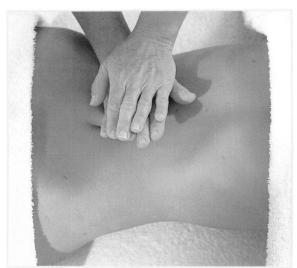

4 With all your fingers pointing in the same direction, create a wavy motion by gently pushing away with the heel of your hand, then pull back with the fingers. Work in a clockwise circle around the belly or move in lines up and down the belly. ◁◁ Repeat step 1. Slowly bring this movement to an end and then rest your hands on the belly for a few seconds, before gently lifting them off.

Now cover your partner's abdomen and move to sit by the head.

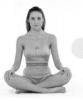

The face

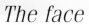

5 Press upwards, underneath and around the cheek bones using your thumbs. Push the weight of your head down on to your thumbs. Press out towards the ears.

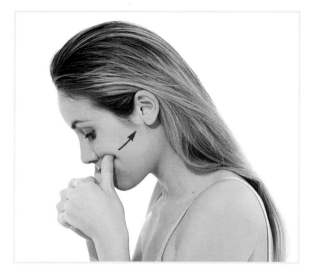

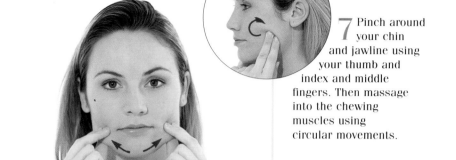

7 Pinch around your chin and jawline using your thumb and index and middle fingers. Then massage into the chewing muscles using circular movements.

48

6 Squeeze the lobes of your ears between your index fingers and thumbs, then work upwards and pull the tops. Now massage the bony area behind the ears using your fingers in small circular movements.

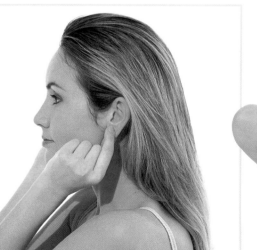

8 Now use the backs of your hands to alternately stroke upwards from the base of the collar bones to the chin. Then stretch the left hand out horizontally under the chin and bounce your right hand up and down slapping against the chin and left hand.

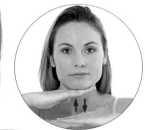

The chest

Avoid massaging over breasts

Ask your partner if she wants her chest area massaged. If not, keep her breasts covered and do steps 3–5

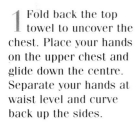

1 Fold back the top towel to uncover the chest. Place your hands on the upper chest and glide down the centre. Separate your hands at waist level and curve back up the sides.

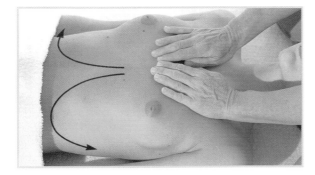

2 Glide down once more. Separate your fingers as you pull your hands apart and feel for the grooves in between the ribs. Do this a few times from the centre working outwards and upwards towards the collar bone.

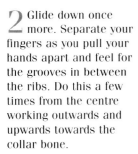
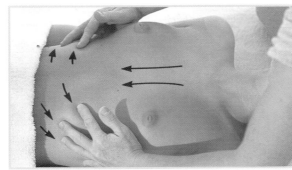
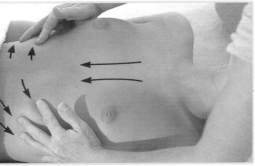

3 On the breast area at the top inner crease of each arm are the pectoral muscles. Knead them lightly with your fingers and thumbs. Work on one side at a time using both hands, then work on both sides simultaneously with one hand on each side.

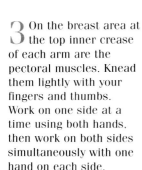
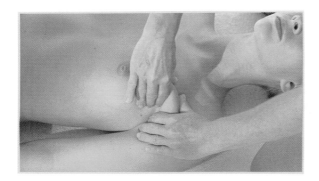

4 Place your hands flat on the upper chest, fingers pointing towards each other. Pull the heels of your hands apart and press down lightly on the shoulders. Curve your hands over and under the shoulders, up the back of the neck and off the head.

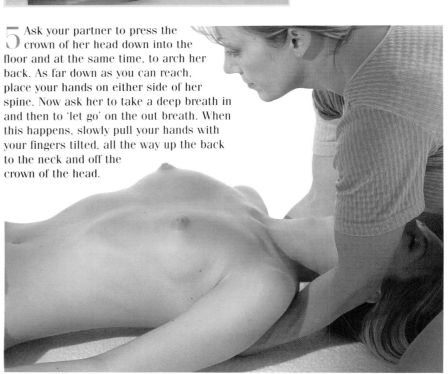

5 Ask your partner to press the crown of her head down into the floor and at the same time, to arch her back. As far down as you can reach, place your hands on either side of her spine. Now ask her to take a deep breath in and then to 'let go' on the out breath. When this happens, slowly pull your hands with your fingers tilted, all the way up the back to the neck and off the crown of the head.

32

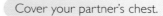

Cover your partner's chest.

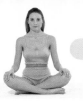

The face

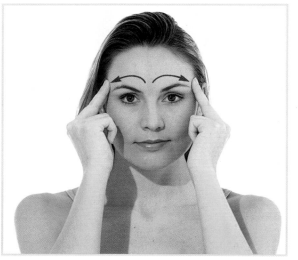

1 Kneel or sit. Place your index and middle fingers above the bridge of your nose. Push upwards to the hairline, then separate your hands and slide out towards the temples. Use small circular movements. Repeat this process, but part the fingers at a lower point each time, until you have worked across the whole forehead.

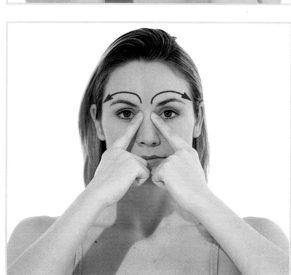

2 Massage the area between the eyebrows to help prevent frownlines. Use your fingers to push upwards and outwards.

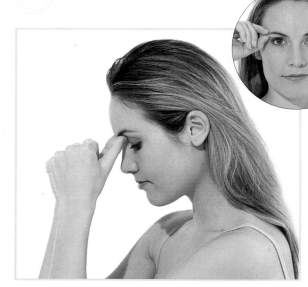

3 Place the pads of your thumbs underneath the inner end of each eyebrow. Press upwards for a few seconds. Now pinch each eyebrow between your index finger and thumb, working outwards.

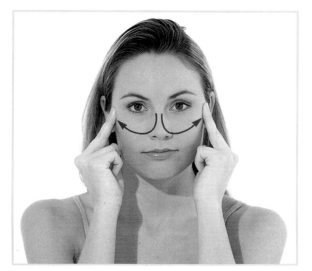

4 Stroke down your nose to the tip, then down the sides and out towards the ears.

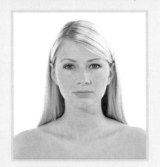

THE NECK, HEAD AND FACE

Massaging the neck, head and face is an excellent way of relieving tension, headaches and anxiety. Massaging the scalp increases circulation to the area and helps to improve the health of the hair.

The neck stretches should be performed very carefully with guidance from your partner as to what feels comfortable.

The tiny facial muscles, not surprisingly, hold a lot of tension as they have to frown, smile, chew and so on all day. A face massage can revitalize your whole body.

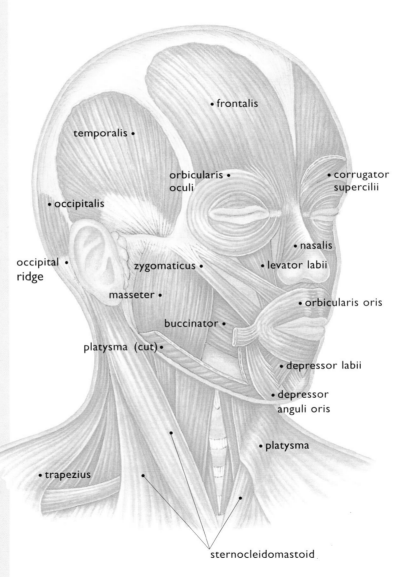

- frontalis
- temporalis •
- orbicularis • oculi
- corrugator supercilii
- occipitalis
- occipital • ridge
- nasalis
- zygomaticus •
- levator labii
- masseter •
- orbicularis oris
- buccinator •
- platysma (cut)•
- depressor labii
- depressor anguli oris
- platysma
- trapezius
- sternocleidomastoid

◀ The skull
Muscles covering the skull, such as frontalis and temporalis, may not be involved in vigorous movement but nevertheless do store some tension and benefit from massage.

◀ The occipital ridge
At the base of the skull along this ridge there are many pressure points. During a neck massage, as you cradle the head, push your fingers and thumbs into these points and hold for 7–10 seconds. This will release blocked energy and tension, as well as feeling extremely pleasant to your partner.

◀ The jaw muscles
The main jaw muscle, masseter, stores a lot of tension particularly in people who clench their jaws.

◀ The facial muscles
Frontalis, corrugator supercilii, orbicularis oris, zygomaticus and depressor anguli oris are all involved in making facial expressions.

◀ The neck muscles
The muscles at the back and sides of the neck – trapezius and sternocleidomastoid – store a lot of tension and may be squeezed with medium pressure. Both these muscles benefit from neck stretches.

33

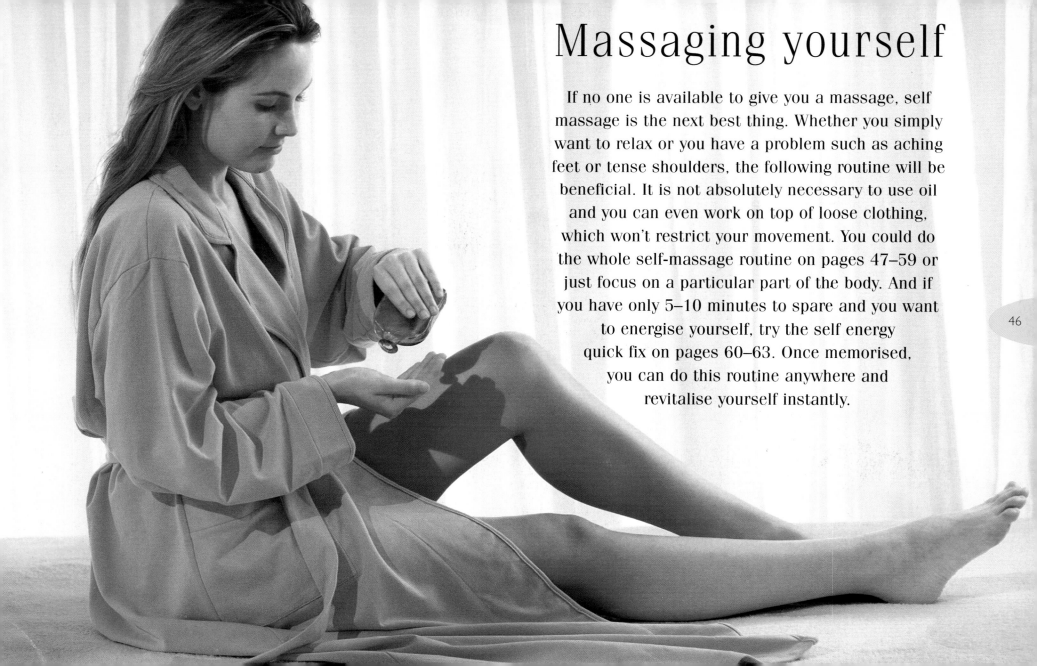

Massaging yourself

If no one is available to give you a massage, self
massage is the next best thing. Whether you simply
want to relax or you have a problem such as aching
feet or tense shoulders, the following routine will be
beneficial. It is not absolutely necessary to use oil
and you can even work on top of loose clothing,
which won't restrict your movement. You could do
the whole self-massage routine on pages 47–59 or
just focus on a particular part of the body. And if
you have only 5–10 minutes to spare and you want
to energise yourself, try the self energy
quick fix on pages 60–63. Once memorised,
you can do this routine anywhere and
revitalise yourself instantly.

The neck

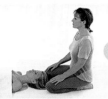

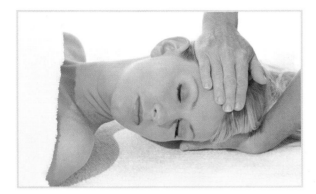

1 Slide your hands underneath the neck and up to the sides of the head. With your hands above the ears lift the head slightly and slowly turn it to face the right side, then turn it to the left.

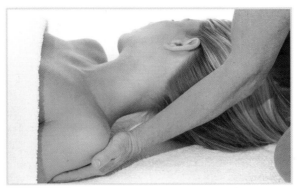

2 Turn the head to the right and let it rest on your right hand. With your left palm, massage in a half moon shape under the back, from the shoulder up to the neck.

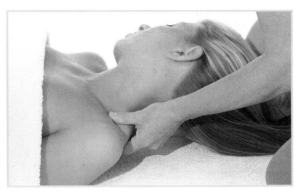

3 Use your thumb and fingers to knead and pinch across the fleshy part at the top of the shoulder. With your fingers press into the back of the shoulder where tension is often stored.

34

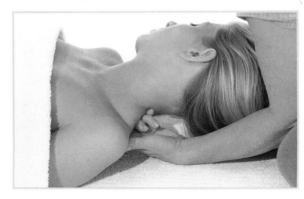

4 Curl your fingertips over and with the flat middle parts, press and rotate them under the shoulder and in towards the base of the neck.

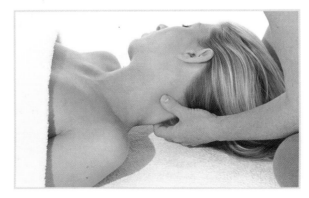

5 Slide your fingers in and under the neck. In a circular movement massage along the relaxed muscles on the right side with your fingers.

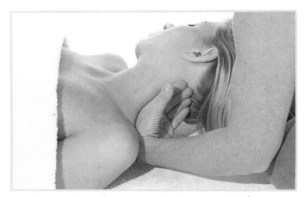

6 Place the back of your hand against the top of the shoulder, fingers pointing inwards. With one long connecting stroke, glide along the shoulder and up the side into the nape of the neck.

◁◁ Repeat steps 1–6 to work on the other side of the neck.

Sitting massage

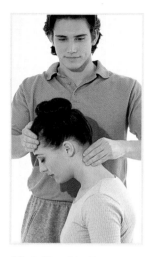

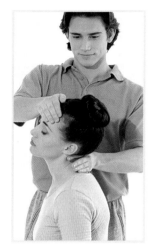

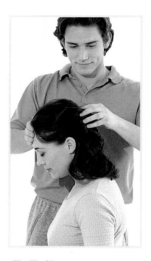

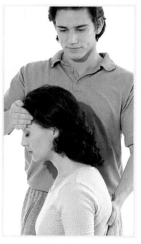

21 Stand to the right side of your partner and place your right hand on her forehead. Ask her to lean her head forwards slightly into your hand and to rest the weight of it there. Bring your left hand up to her neck. Knead up and down with your thumb and fingers in a circular motion. Massage the whole of the neck area.

22 Keep supporting her head with your right hand. Open your left thumb and fingers and bring your hand underneath the bony ridge at the base of the skull. Tilt her head back slightly, but not too far or you'll strain her neck. Roll her head towards the left and on to the end of your index finger. Now slowly roll the head back to the right towards the end of your thumb. Roll the head a few times then squeeze under the ridge.

23 Keep supporting her head with your right hand. If your partner's hair was tied back, loosen it now. Massage upwards with your fingers as if shampooing the hair. Change hands and support the head from underneath while you massage the top, stroking up and over the forehead to finish. ◁◁ Repeat steps 21, 22 and 23 from the other side.

24 Move to the right again and support her head in your right hand as before. Bring your left hand to the centre of your partner's back at the base of the shoulder blades. Remain still for about 30 seconds. Slowly release your hand from the back. Bring your partner's head up and remove your right hand.

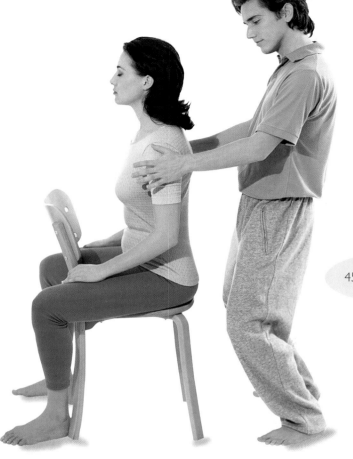

25 Stand behind your partner and brush down the tops of her shoulders and arms. Repeat a few times before brushing down the whole of her back, bringing your massage to a close. This gives a cleansing, refreshing feeling to revive your partner at the end of the massage.

45

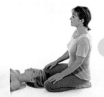

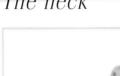

The neck

Avoid if your partner has a neck problem

7 Stroke up the neck from the base a few times, alternating your hands. Then curl your fingers and press them into the bony ridge at the base of the skull. Rest the backs of the hands on the floor and cradle the head in this position for approximately 30 seconds.

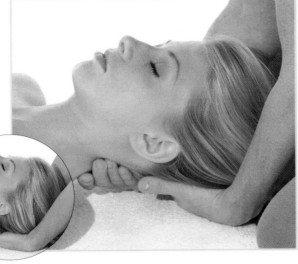

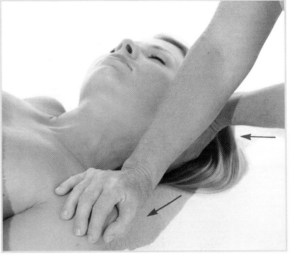

9 Still using both hands, lift your partner's head and move her right ear down towards her right shoulder. Place your left hand on the side of the head, then cross your right hand over and place it against your partner's left shoulder. Now gently push your hands in opposite directions.

35

8 Place your flat hands under the head. Lift the head slightly and gently pull backwards. Now lift the head higher and push against it so that the chin moves towards the chest. This stretches the back of the neck. Lower the head.

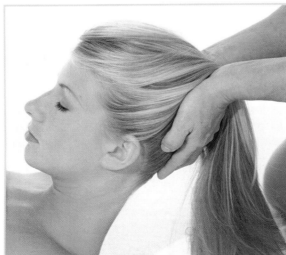

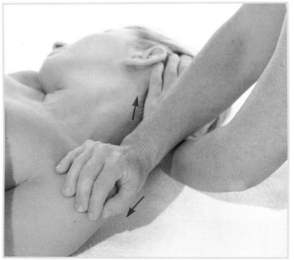

10 Uncross your hands and turn your partner's head so that her nose now points towards her right shoulder. Cross your hands and place the heel of your left hand under the bony ridge at the base of her skull. Rest your right hand on top of her left shoulder. Push your hands gently in opposite directions. Uncross your hands and straighten your partner's head.

◁◁ Repeat steps 9 and 10 on the opposite side.

Sitting massage

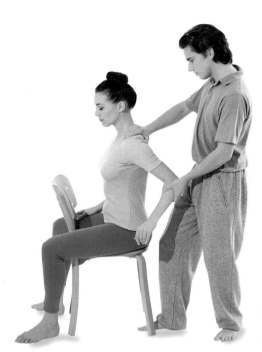

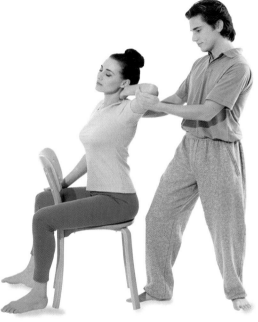

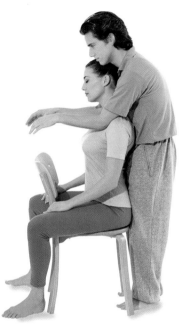

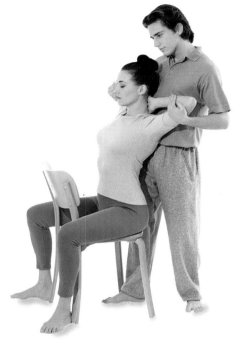

44

17 Rest your right hand flat on your partner's shoulder. Move forwards and grasp her left arm just below the elbow. Rotate the arm forwards and up in a circular motion, as you gently push forwards against the shoulder with your right hand. Move your left foot forwards as you do this, to keep your weight even on both legs. Rotate the arm a few times before flowing into the next step.

18 As you rotate the arm up, bend your partner's elbow so that her hand rests behind her head. Push forwards on the back of her right shoulder as you pull back the top of the left arm to stretch the chest. Do not use too much force – ask your partner how far this stretch is comfortable. Lower the arm.
◁◁ Repeat steps 17 and 18 on the other side.

19 Bring your forearms over your partner's shoulders. Bend your elbows and press them in above her chest, while pulling back with your shoulders to stretch her chest. At the same time, push your body forwards into her back to support it.

20 Grasp both your partner's forearms just below the elbows and bring them up above her head. Ask your partner to clasp her hands together behind her head and inhale. Bring your hands underneath and around her forearms and pull them back as your partner exhales. Push your pelvis into her back to support it as you pull her arms back. Repeat, then lower your partner's arms.

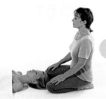

The head

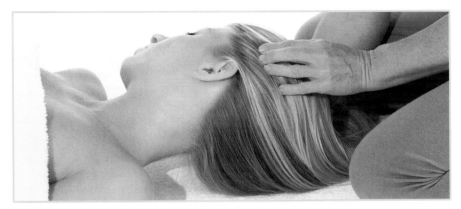

1 Slide your hands underneath the neck and up to the sides of the head, with your thumbs around the ears. Gently turn the head to the right and work on the left half. With your left hand massage the scalp in circles against the skull.

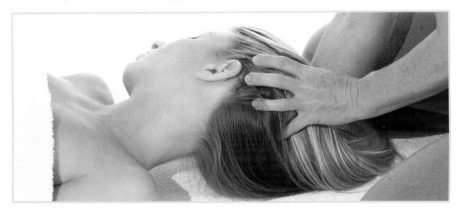

2 With your fingers spread apart and bent, use the tips to rub into your partner's scalp as if shampooing her hair. Make sure that you work underneath the head as well as on the side.

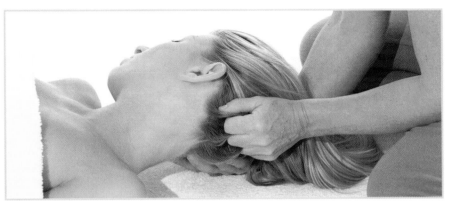

3 With your left hand, grab handfuls of hair close to the roots and pull firmly to stimulate the roots. Gently turn the head to the left. ◁◁ Repeat steps 1–3 on the right side.

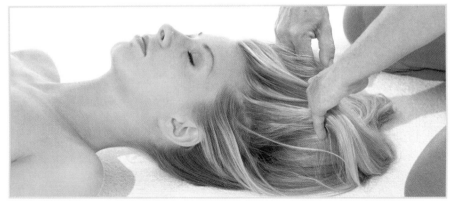

4 Straighten the head. Stroke your palms over the forehead and up over the top of the head. Open your fingers and comb through the hair, first on the top then out to the sides and back to the top.

Sitting massage

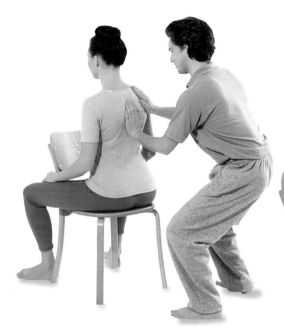

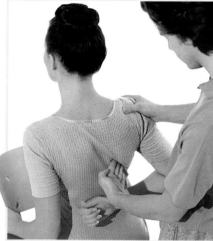

43

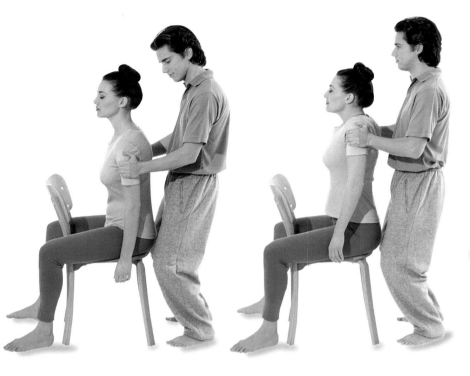

13 Remove the cushion. Ask your partner to sit upright again. Work on one shoulder blade at a time. Rub up and down across the blade with flat hands. Rub in towards the muscles next to the spine. Then with open fingers grab and lift the muscles over the blade.

14 Bend your partner's right elbow, and bring her forearm behind her back. Bring your right hand around the front of her right shoulder over the joint. Straighten the fingers of your left hand and push them under the blade at an angle, as you pull the shoulder towards you. Work all around the inner side of the blade using your fingers and thumb. Return your partner's arm to a relaxed position. ◁◁ Repeat steps 13 and 14 on the other side.

15 Let your partner's arms hang by her sides. Then squeeze down the arms from the shoulders to the wrists using both your hands. Repeat a few times, covering the front, back and sides of her arms.

16 Grasp the tops of both arms. Ask your partner to breathe in as you lift her shoulders up and around her ears. Hold for a few seconds and then let go while telling her to exhale. Repeat a few times.

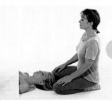

The face

 Use a very small amount of oil if necessary

 Make sure your partner has removed contact lenses

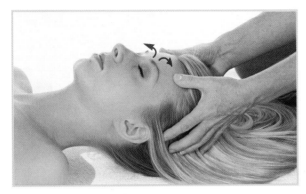

1 Place your thumbs just above the centre of the eyebrows and press out to the temples. Repeat this, working in lines, until you have covered the whole of the forehead.

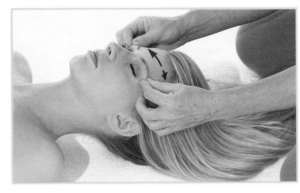

2 Using your thumbs and index fingers lightly pinch underneath and on top of the eyebrows from the centre outwards. Repeat several times.

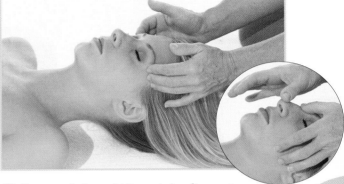

3 Use your index, middle and ring fingers to massage in small circular movements around the temples and sides of the head. Do not press too hard. Then use alternate thumbs to stroke down the nose.

37

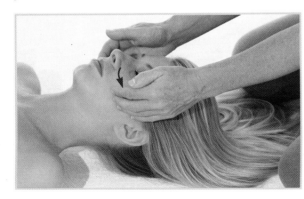

4 With fingers together massage from the nose along the cheek to the ear. Move your fingers slightly down and repeat. Work in lines to cover the cheek area, following the contours of the face.

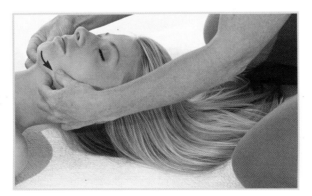

5 Then pinch along the chin and jawbone with your thumbs and index fingers. Finally, with the flat of your fingers, using circular movements, work into the muscles of the jaw.

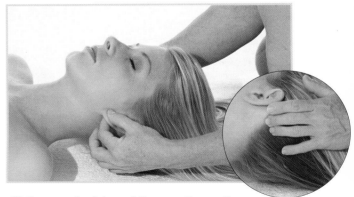

6 Squeeze the lobes of the ears then pull and squeeze all around the ears, up to the tops and back again. Now use your middle fingers to massage the bony ridge behind the ears.

Sitting massage

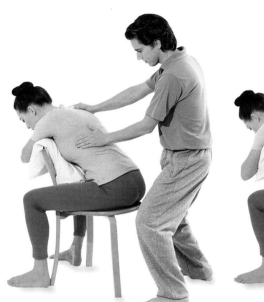
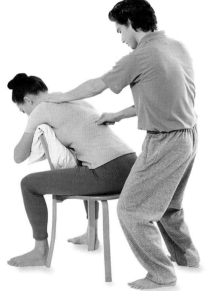
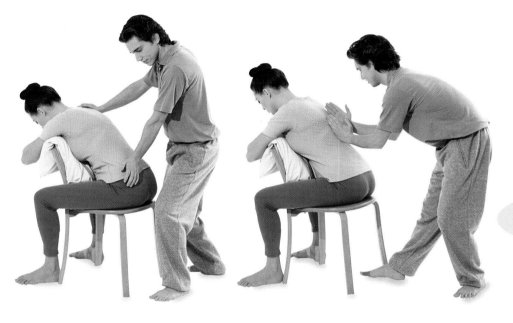

9 Place a cushion over the back of the chair. Ask your partner to lean forward. Rub the left side of the back with your left palm, keeping it flat. Then make a fist and rub the left side of the back. Work into the lower back and push down into the buttocks. Change hands and repeat on the other side.

10 Rest your left hand on your partner's left shoulder. Bend the index finger of your right hand in half. Starting level with the middle of the shoulder blades, use your thumb and bent finger on either side of the spine, to exert static pressure for about 7 seconds at a time, working down to the base of the spine. Change hands and repeat.

11 Rest your right hand on your partner's right shoulder. Use the heel of your left hand to push down and into the lower back. Then press along the tops of the buttocks with your thumb. Change hands and repeat.

12 Using the sides of your hands, place them on either side of the spine, at the top of the back. Rub them backwards and forwards about 5 cm in opposite directions. Now use this technique up and down the entire length of the spine.

42

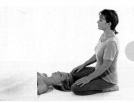

Connecting the face and head

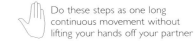
Do these steps as one long continuous movement without lifting your hands off your partner

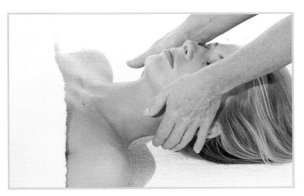

1 Slide your fingers under the neck and then bring the heels of your hands up onto the cheeks, push them down and out to the ears.

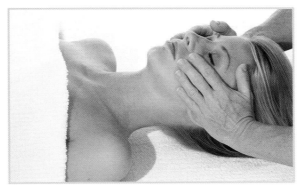

2 Twist your fingers back and up, resting your fingers at the sides of the nose. Slide them apart and down to the ears.

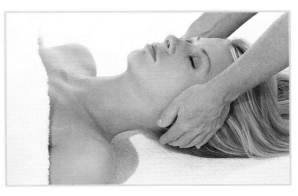

3 Twist your fingers down and cup your hands over the ears. Remain still for a few seconds, closing out all sounds.

38

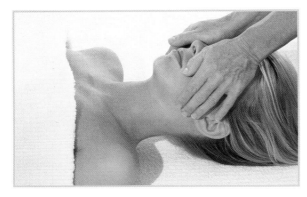

4 Bring your palms up and cup your hands over the eyes. Remain still again for a few seconds, blocking out the light.

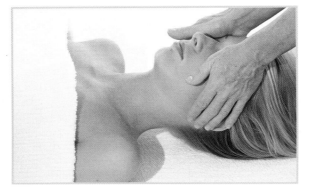

5 Part your hands slowly. Then using the muscles at the base of your thumbs brush lightly across the eyelids and out to the temples.

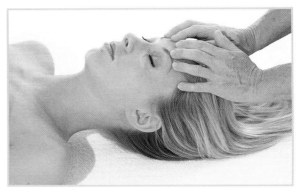

6 Twist your fingers up and onto the eyebrows and then pull the fingers up and over the forehead and comb them through the hair.

Sitting massage

Avoid step 7 if your partner is pregnant

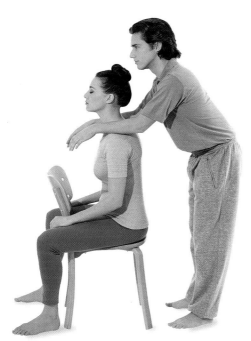
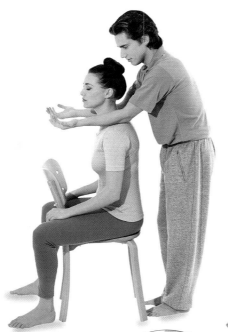
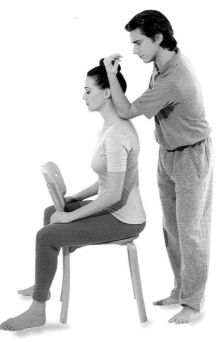
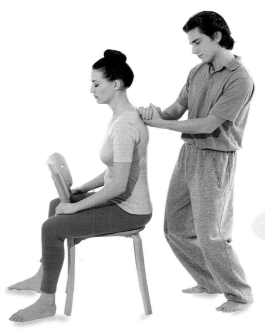

41

5 Place your forearms on top of your partner's shoulders with your palms facing down. Use your body weight to push them down alternately. Be gentle at first, then gradually add more pressure. Ask your partner how much pressure is comfortable.

6 With your forearms still on top of your partner's shoulders, press down and roll them apart, turning your palms upwards as you do so. Repeat, then roll your arms alternately with one palm facing up, one down so that pressure is applied to the shoulders alternately.

7 Rest your right hand on top of your partner's right shoulder. Now bring your left elbow to rest on the high point of her left shoulder, near to the neck. Relax your wrist and hand as you press down with your elbow. Work outwards toward the middle of the shoulder. Repeat on the other side.

8 Clasp your hands together and use the back of one of them to hit across the back of the shoulders and upper back. You should hear the air escaping between your palms.

Connecting the body

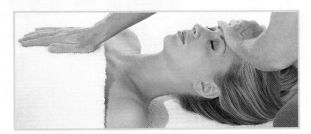

1 Place your left hand gently across your partner's forehead and your right hand on her chest, fingers pointing to her feet. Stay completely still for a few seconds. Watch your partner's breathing and as she breathes in, lightly lift your hands off.

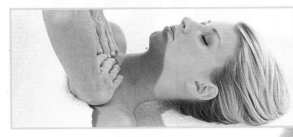

2 Move to your partner's right side. With your fingers pointing towards one another place your hands on the upper chest. Move your hands out to the shoulders, down each arm and off the hands.

3 Place your hands back on the chest, with your fingers facing upwards. Move them down between the breasts, then out and over the hips, trace over the tops of the legs and then off the toes.

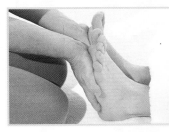

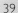

4 Sitting at the feet, place the palms of your hands against the soles of the feet. Then slide your hands under the heels and gently pull them towards you.

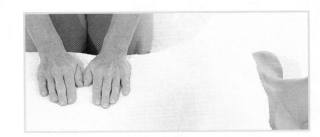

5 Move to your partner's right side, facing in and rest both hands on her belly. Remain in this position for about one minute. Then lightly lift your hands off. Allow your partner to rest quietly and enjoy inner peace and tranquillity.

39

Sitting massage

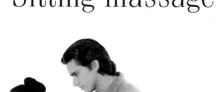

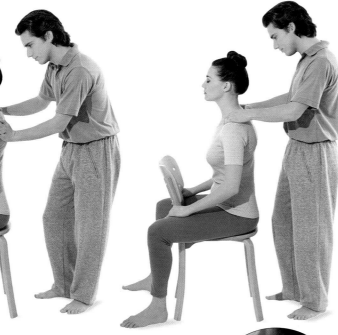

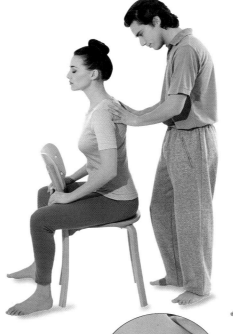

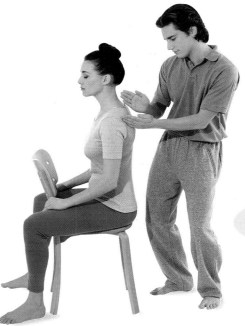

40

1 Ask your partner to sit upright on a chair, facing the back of it. Stand behind her and rub your hands together above your head for about one minute. Now rest your hands on your partner's shoulders as you relax and breathe deeply. Allow the warmth of your hands to penetrate into your partner, remaining still for 30 seconds. Using flat palms, rub across the top of your partner's shoulders, then down, around and on top of the shoulder blades.

2 Using both hands, knead and squeeze into the muscles at the tops of the shoulders. Then grasp the muscles and lift them, as if pulling them up away from the bones.

3 Place your thumbs on either side of the spine and knead into the muscles using circular movements. Work down to the base of the spine.

4 Place your hands on the shoulders, grasp the muscles and 'shake' them. Then, with loose wrists and fingers, use the sides of your hands in a 'karate chop' action to hack across the tops and backs of the shoulders.

GLOSSARY

BACK HAND SLAPPING A percussion technique using the back of the hands to slap against the flesh.

CATERPILLAR WALK A technique where the thumb is alternately bent and straightened, moving as if it was a caterpillar. Useful along the arch of the foot.

CONNECTING Bringing together the energy of various parts of the body.

CUPPING A percussion technique where the hands are cupped as if to scoop water and are used to drum against the flesh.

DEEP MUSCLES Those muscles that lie beneath superficial muscles.

DRAGON'S MOUTH POSITION A technique used on the legs. The fingers are kept together and spread apart from the thumb to form a V-shape – then push over the knee and lower leg.

EFFLEURAGE This is the French word for 'stroking' and is done all over the body at the beginning of a massage to warm and prepare the muscles for deeper pressure, and at the end of a massage to relax the muscles.

ESSENTIAL OILS Oils extracted from the parts of aromatic plants. They have various properties which can be therapeutic for both physical and emotional problems.

HACKING A percussion technique where the sides of the hands are used to 'karate chop' the flesh rapidly.

KNEADING A deep tissue technique used over very fleshy parts of the body like the buttocks and shoulders. The hands alternately squeeze and push the flesh as if wringing out a wet cloth or kneading dough.

LYMPH The fluid containing white blood cells, fats and proteins, which filters out of the bloodstream, accumulates in body tissues and then enters the lymphatic vessels.

LYMPHATIC SYSTEM Vessels, nodes (glands) and organs which help to maintain the correct fluid balance in blood and tissues as well as being responsible for the body's immune function.

LYMPHATIC DRAINAGE A massage technique to improve the removal of wastes and excess fluid from the body.

MERIDIANS A network of energy channels which are connected to organs and run throughout the body.

PERCUSSION Brisk bouncy movements used on fleshy, muscular parts of the body. Should not be used over bony areas, bruises or varicose veins.

PETRISSAGE A medium pressure technique where the flesh is pushed against underlying bone. Includes thumb circling and thumb rolling.

PLUCKING A percussion technique where the fingers are used to pinch and pluck the flesh.

PRESSURE POINTS An opening into the meridian where energy can be reached and influenced, with specific healing reactions upon the body and mind.

PUMMELLING A percussion technique where the hands form loose fists and drum rapidly against the flesh.

ROCKING Gently pushing the body to relax it.

REFLEXES A term in reflexology to describe areas within ten longitudinal zones of the feet, corresponding to divisions in the body.

SUPERFICIAL MUSCLES Those muscles just below the skin and its underlying fat.

VENOUS FLOW The flow of the blood through the veins back to the heart.

ACKNOWLEDGEMENTS

Carroll & Brown would very much like to thank:

Dr Amanda Roberts for checking anatomy illustrations

Peggy Sadler and Mercedes Morgan for additional design work

Paul Williams for arrow illustrations

Nadia Silver for editorial assistance

Jo Stanford for the index

Bettina Graham for hair and make-up

Margaret-Ann Hugo and Mark Langridge for photography assistance

Dorian Cassidy for administrative assistance

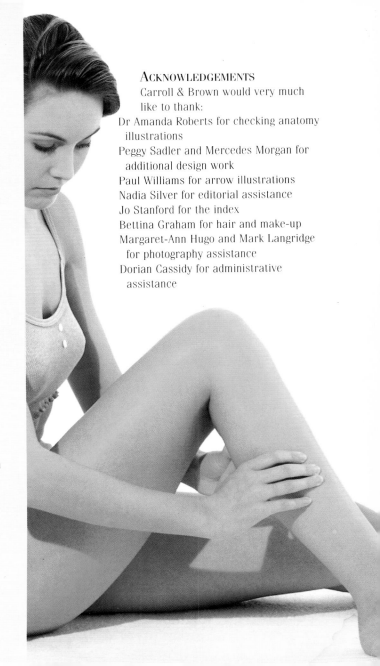

INDEX